FLOW &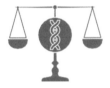
THRIVE

How to Boost Your Health with Lymphatic Drainage is a practical guide that helps you unlock the secrets of your body's lymphatic system, empowering you to achieve balance and optimal health.

by Summer Maiden, LMT, NMT

Flow & Thrive

How to Boost your Health with Lymphatic Drainage

For permission requests, contact the author/self-publisher at:
Summer Maiden, LMT, NMT
Email/www.waze2wellness.com

Book and Cover design by Summer Maiden, LMT, NMT

Disclaimer: This book is intended for informational purposes only. It is not a substitute for professional medical advice, diagnosis, or treatment. Always seek the advice of your physician or qualified health provider with any questions you may have regarding a medical condition.

ISBN: 979-8-9917720-0-6

First Edition 2024

Printed in the United States of America

TABLE OF CONTENTS

ACKNOWLEGEMENTS

Writing a book is never a solitary endeavor, and I am grateful to the many individuals whose support and encouragement have made this journey possible.

First and foremost, I would like to express my deepest gratitude to God for his wisdom and knowledge and to my family and closest friends for their unwavering love, support, and encouragement throughout this process. Your belief in me has been my greatest source of strength.

I want to extend my appreciation to my editor, Leslie Poteet Busker, for her expertise and dedication in bringing this book to life. Your professionalism and passion for excellence have made this collaboration truly rewarding.

INTRODUCTION

The human body is a marvel of biological engineering, and the lymphatic system is one of its most crucial yet often overlooked components. This system is responsible for filtering out toxins, maintaining fluid balance, and supporting the immune system. Over the last few years, lymphatic drainage has gained popularity as a holistic therapy aimed at improving the function of the lymphatic system. This eBook explores the benefits of lymphatic drainage, the science behind it, and how it can contribute to overall health and well-being.

By understanding the importance of the lymphatic system and the science behind lymphatic drainage, individuals can make well-informed decisions about incorporating this therapy into their wellness routines. Whether seeking relief from chronic conditions or simply looking to enhance overall health, Lymphatic Drainage Massage can be a valuable addition to a holistic health regimen.

A LETTER FROM THE AUTHOR

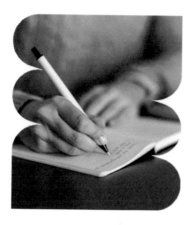

As a Licensed Massage Therapist since 2006, I have been doing manual Lymphatic Drainage Massage since the beginning. I was inspired by a colleague of mine, whom I followed during my rotations while employed at the hospital as a medical massage therapist. The results my colleague was getting with the patients using the lymphatic drainage modality truly amazed me. I knew this was how I wanted to start my career. I have now practiced this treatment in multiple hospital environments, including General Health, Hematology/Oncology, Cardiac, Pulmonary, Post-Surgery, Pregnancy, and Rehabilitation. Currently, due to the rising interest from my clients who became curious about adding this particular modality to their health journey, I decided to write this book.

THANK YOU

Thank you for choosing Flow & Thrive: How to Boost Your Health with Lymphatic Drainage. Your decision to explore and invest in your well-being through this content means a lot to me. I hope the insights and information provided enrich your journey toward a healthier, more balanced life. For more from the Waze2Wellness platform, visit our store.

Store: www.waze2wellnes.store
email: waze2wellness@gmail.com

In good health,

Summer Maiden

CHAPTER ONE

UNDERSTANDING
THE LYMPHATIC SYSTEM

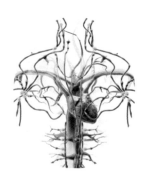

What is the Lymphatic System? The lymphatic system is a one-way system that is composed of a network of organs and tissues that help rid the body of toxins, waste, and other unwanted materials. It is designed to maintain fluid balance and enhance the natural flow of lymph fluid throughout the body, promoting immune function, detoxification, and overall wellness. Interestingly, it is a component of the circulatory system. Lymph does not move in a circuit or a circle, though. Lymph flows in the direction of the cardiovascular system. Lymph does not have a centralized pump such as the heart does with the cardiovascular system. Instead, it moves along with the pull of gravity and without the aid of the heart's direct pumping action. It also relies on external forces like deep breathing and physical movements such as muscle contractions, causing a squeeze and release action that exerts pressure on the lymphatic vessel walls.

Other forces that promote flow are pulsing actions of nearby large arteries such as the aorta, postural changes, and compressive forces such as massage, the application of bandages, and hydrostatic pressure from water activities such as swimming. Both systems, the lymphatic and the circulatory, transport pathogenic substances, foreign bodies, and large proteins. Thus, both systems act on our behalf as a purification system by breaking down and destroying particles that need to be eliminated from the body.

What is the Lymphatic System? The lymphatic system is a one-way system that is composed of a network of organs and tissues that help rid the body of toxins, waste, and other unwanted materials. It is designed to maintain fluid balance and enhance the natural flow of lymph fluid throughout the body, promoting immune function, detoxification, and overall wellness. Interestingly, it is a component of the circulatory system. Lymph does not move in a circuit or a circle, though. Lymph flows in the direction of the cardiovascular system. Lymph does not have a centralized pump such as the heart does with the cardiovascular system. Instead, it moves along with the pull of gravity and without the aid of the heart's direct pumping action. It also relies on external forces like deep breathing and physical movements such as muscle contractions, causing a squeeze and release action that exerts pressure on the lymphatic vessel walls. Other forces that promote flow are pulsing actions of nearby large arteries such as the aorta, postural changes, and compressive forces such as massage, the application of bandages, and hydrostatic pressure from water activities such as swimming.

Both systems, the lymphatic and the circulatory, transport pathogenic substances, foreign bodies, and large proteins. Thus, both systems act on our behalf as a purification system by breaking down and destroying particles that need to be eliminated from the body.

Key lymphatic system organs consist of bone marrow, the thymus, the spleen, and the liver. Other components are lymph, lymph nodes, lymphocytes, and lymph vessels, which we will discuss in detail later. All play a crucial role in maintaining fluid balance, removing toxins, and supporting immune responses. When the toxic contents of the lymphatic system move, the pressure generated stimulates lymph flow, which encourages the removal of excess fluid and waste products and promotes circulation to reduce swelling and inflammation.

By, improving the efficiency of this essential system can have a profound effect on our health's vitality. If our lymphatic system does not absorb the toxic contents that escape from interstitial fluid, the body would likely develop significant edema (swelling) and autointoxication (automatic toxicity) that could cause death within 1-2 days (Guyton).

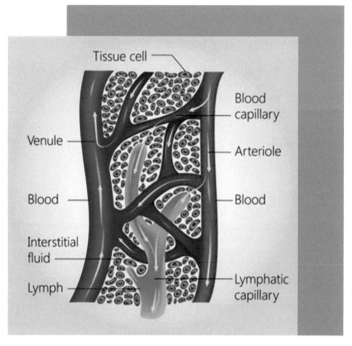

*This illustration shows the
arteriole, venous and lymphatic flow*

Regarding location, the lymphatic system is present everywhere in the body except in tissues where there is no blood cell development and in types of tissue that drain directly from the body. These areas include 1) epithelial tissue(epidermis), cartilage, and the cornea and lens of the eye, and 2) the placenta, passageways of the inner ear, and structures of the central nervous system, respectively. Now let's take a further look at each of the key components of the lymphatic system.

Key Parts of our Lymphatic System:

Lymph: A clear interstitial fluid that is very important. It contains white blood cells, which are crucial for fighting infections. The elements of lymph include water, lipids (fat), free cells, proteins, enzymes, minerals, hormones, cells, and toxins, to name a few. As a comparison, lymph contains more water than blood plasma does. It is 96% water. Lymph fluid maintains and regulates the fluid ratio between the blood and the tissues.

The lymph fluid receives nutrients and rejects damaged products. Simplified, once this fluid is inside the connective tissues of the body and enters the lymph capillaries, it's then called lymph. Our lymphatic system is made in such a way that it fine-tunes the drainage process, keeping it from creating an overflow and allowing it to evacuate water and excess substances from the interstitial environment.

Before we go further, I would like to define a few important parts of lymph fluid:

Lipids: Lipids recuperate the fat absorbed during digestion in the intestinal tract, mainly free fatty acids and lipoproteins.

The Free Cells: These free cells are part of the lymph flow; they vary and multiply when going through lymph nodes or when infectious tissue is present.

The Proteins: The proteins help with a very important lymphatic function by recirculating the proteins that have leaked from blood circulation. Massive swelling will occur if the lymphatic system does not recover these proteins.

Lymph is the only system in the body that can regain trapped excess proteins. These proteins can become restricted within tissues due to various factors, including limited physical activity, low oxygen levels, inadequate nutrition, the buildup of environmental and metabolic toxins, high-stress levels, and the natural aging process.

The lymph system moves these proteins out of the tissues through specialized lymphatic channels, filtering and eventually returning them to the bloodstream. The lymphatic system supports optimal circulation, immune health, and homeostasis by maintaining lymph fluid balance and protein regulation.

The Hormones: Lymph also significantly impacts hormone balance and function. Hormones, chemical messengers released by glands in the endocrine system, rely on efficient circulation to reach target tissues throughout the body. The lymphatic system not only helps transport hormones but also aids in clearing away excess hormones and metabolic byproducts, preventing imbalances. When the lymphatic system is sluggish or congested due to factors like inactivity, stress, or toxin buildup, hormones can accumulate or struggle to reach their destinations effectively.

This congestion can lead to hormonal imbalances, influencing everything from stress response (cortisol) to mood (serotonin, dopamine) and reproductive health (estrogen, progesterone). The lymphatic system supports a stable internal environment by consistently removing waste products and excess hormones, promoting balanced hormone production and function.

Additionally, the lymph system supports the immune system, which is closely linked to endocrine health. Chronic inflammation or immune issues, often arising from a compromised lymphatic system, can disrupt hormone levels and lead to long-term effects like adrenal fatigue, thyroid issues, or reproductive hormone imbalances. In this way, a healthy, active lymphatic system plays a critical role in maintaining hormonal equilibrium.

The Toxins: Toxins within the lymph are unwanted substances, like waste products, environmental pollutants, and byproducts of cellular metabolism, that the body needs to remove to stay healthy. These toxins can enter the body through things we eat, breathe, and absorb through the skin, as well as from natural metabolic processes. The lymphatic system collects these waste materials from tissues throughout the body and transports them to lymph nodes, which act as "filtering stations." Inside the lymph nodes, white blood cells work to break down and neutralize these toxins. Once the toxins are processed in the lymph nodes, they are moved toward the bloodstream, where the body can eliminate them through the liver, kidneys, and skin. This cleansing process helps prevent toxin buildup that could otherwise lead to inflammation, fatigue, and a weakened immune system.

Lymph Nodes: Lymph nodes are small bean-shaped structures that filter lymph and store white blood cells. A normal healthy size lymph node ranges from 2mm to 25 mm. Our bodies contain between 400 and 700 of these nodes. Over half are located in the abdomen, while many more are found in the cervical/neck region. Also, the main groups of nodes are located in the major articulation folds (e.g., the back of the knee).

The lymph nodes are part of the lymphoid system, which comprises various tissues and organs and is part of the immune system. The lymphoid system produces and/or carries lymphocytes and related cells.

Lymph Nodes have various functions:
- filtration and purification for lymph circulation
- capture and destroy toxins
- concentrate the lymph
- produce lymphocytes (when lymph flow increases)

Lymphocytes: Lymphocytes are a type of white blood cell. They help your body's immune system fight cancer, foreign viruses, and bacteria. As a vital part of your immune system, your lymphocytes aid in protecting you from infections as well as aid in destroying old or abnormal cells your body doesn't need. This helps to maintain normal fluid levels and to absorb fats and fat-soluble vitamins so they can make their way into your bloodstream.

Lymph Vessels: Lymph vessels are a network of tubes that transport lymph throughout the body.

Spleen, Thymus, and Tonsils: These are organs that play a role in the production and maturation of lymphocytes.

LYMPHATIC SYSTEM

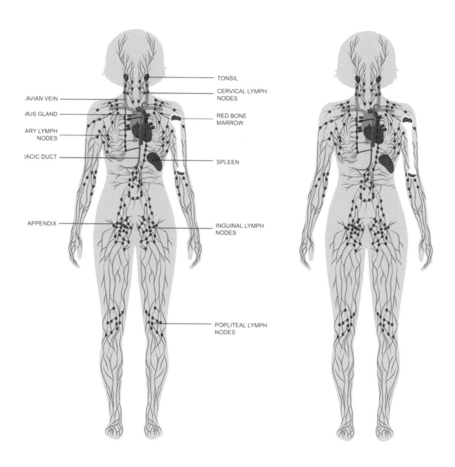

TONSIL

CERVICAL LYMPH
NODES

AVIAN VEIN

MUS GLAND

RED BONE
MARROW

ARY LYMPH
NODES

ACIC DUCT

SPLEEN

APPENDIX

INGUINAL LYMPH
NODES

POPLITEAL LYMPH
NODES

The Liver: The liver plays a significant, multifaceted role in lymph drainage involving detoxification, immune function, regulation of fluid balance, the production of lymph fluid, and fat metabolism. This is crucial for maintaining overall health and well-being.

The following list details, more specifically, the liver's involvement with the lymph system:

Detoxification: The liver is the body's primary detoxification organ. It filters out toxins from the blood, which are then excreted into the bile and removed from the body. The lymphatic system assists in transporting these filtered substances away from tissues and towards the liver for processing.

Fat Process: The liver processes proteins and fats, which are then transported via the lymphatic system.

Lymphatic Support: By detoxifying the blood, the liver reduces the load of harmful substances that the lymphatic system has to deal with.

Immune Cell Production: The liver produces various immune cells, such as Kupffer cells (a type of cell-eater called a macrophage), which play a crucial role in the body's immune response. These immune cells can be transported through the lymphatic system to sites of infection or injury.

Production: The liver produces a substantial portion of the body's lymph fluid. It is a highly vascular organ, and its blood vessels contribute to the formation of lymph.

Lymphocyte Activation: The liver also contributes to activating and regulating lymphocytes to help defend the body against pathogens.

Regulation of Fluid Balance: The liver produces albumin, a protein that helps maintain osmotic pressure in the blood vessels, ensuring fluid does not excessively leak into tissues. Proper fluid balance is crucial for preventing edema and supporting efficient lymphatic drainage.

Fat Metabolism: The liver processes dietary fats absorbed from the intestines and packages them into lipoproteins. These lipoproteins are then transported through the lymphatic system, allowing fat metabolism to occur.

Issues to consider with the liver: Diseases such as liver cirrhosis or hepatitis can impair the liver's ability to produce lymph and filter toxins, negatively affecting the lymphatic system.

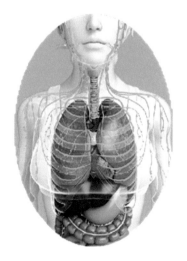

Illustration of the liver, spleen and lymph flow

CHAPTER TWO

THE SCIENCE OF LYMPHATIC DRAINAGE MASSAGE

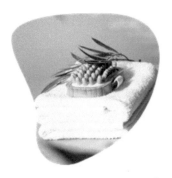

Lymphatic Drainage Massage, also known as MDL (Manual Lymphatic Drainage), is a therapeutic technique that involves gentle, rhythmic massage to stimulate the flow of lymph fluid throughout the body. It is designed to enhance the natural function of the lymphatic system. It can be done anytime and as frequently as you desire. Treatments can be regularly scheduled routine sessions for a general health and wellness lifestyle, simply for various ailments, or post- surgery to reduce fluid and swelling.

By law, a Massage Therapist CANNOT diagnose diseases. However, some disorders are contraindicated for this modality and must be considered by the therapist. Completing a thorough and truthful intake form is crucial.

So, what is Lymphatic Drainage Massage?

Lymphatic Drainage Massage (MLD) is a hands-on technique in which a therapist uses light pressure, rhythmic movements, and pumping to produce peristaltic waves of contractions of the surrounding tissue. This encourages lymph flow and is not correlated to the pulse or breathing. These rhythmic contractions provide efficient action on the circulation of the lymph. When manually stimulated, the capacity of the whole lymphatic system is increased by about 20 times what it is normally able to do on its own.

How Does it Work?

Functionally, the therapist employs a passive, rhythmic pumping-type action to move lymph around the external stretch receptors after they are engaged. In our chest cavity, when the diaphragm's inhalation and exhalation movements occur, the cavity undergoes negative pressure in the abdominal region. This is called the respiratory pump action. For this reason, the therapist will ask you to breathe and/or take deep breaths during the sessions.

Lymphatic Drainage Massage not only assists in regulating fluid volume and pressure but also reduces edema by indirectly dilating blood capillaries, stimulating reabsorption, and activating venous circulation. When our lymph passes into our lymph nodes, it boosts our cellular immunity along with our immune system. Additionally, it affects our nervous system by decreasing the sympathetic response (fight or flight) and stimulates the parasympathetic mode (rest and relaxation).

This lymphatic pump aids in skeletal muscle contractions, peristalsis of the abdomen, contractions of adjacent arteries, and increased mobility of limbs by decreasing the accumulated fluids. When Lymphatic Drainage Massage is performed, the external pressure affects our system, like 1) water when swimming and 2) bandages used for compression. Exercise can stimulate many factors for deep lymphatic circulation, but superficial lymph circulation is not directly affected. Thus, Lymphatic Drainage Massages are particularly beneficial in reducing swelling and edema in superficial circulation within the skin.

The Process and Drainage Effect of Lymphatic Massage:

Treatments allow the therapist to "reroute" stagnant fluid in the skin, mucosa, muscles, abdomen, joints, cranial structures, and eye chambers. When this happens, the removal of toxins promotes tissue regeneration which helps scars from forming dense scar tissue, stretch marks, or the post-surgery scarring condition called fibrosis. Along with this, fluid reabsorption eliminates any protein-rich fluid collected from extracellular tissue eliminating the edema. Whenever fat content is present, lymphatic vessels are also present to help evacuate them.

For the body's immunity, Lymphatic Drainage Massage can increase lymph flow, carrying more antigens to the lymph nodes and increasing antibodies/antigens. This can be useful for chronic or subacute inflammation, chronic fatigue, autoimmune diseases, bronchitis, sinusitis, tonsillitis, laryngitis, arthritis, acne, and many other diagnoses.

When alleviating issues such as fluid stagnation, receptors that trigger pain, muscle spasms, and constipation, and reducing constipation, we stimulate the parasympathetic system, which in turn decreases the sympathetic tone (fight-or-flight response). This can aid significantly with sleeping disorders, depression, and stress.

There can be actual visual indications that Lymphatic Drainage Massage is needed. These indicators include 1) abnormal edema - swelling, and 2) pitted edema -when a fingerprint leaves an indentation. These can be indicators of the system not working correctly, a mechanical insufficiency, and one of the main indicators that Lymphatic Drainage Massage is needed.

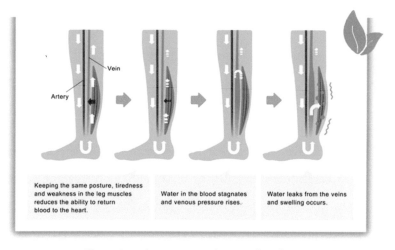

Keeping the same posture, tiredness and weakness in the leg muscles reduces the ability to return blood to the heart.

Water in the blood stagnates and venous pressure rises.

Water leaks from the veins and swelling occurs.

Illustration of stagnation and stages of swelling.

After exploring how manual manipulation of the lymphatic drainage system works, we can realize health and immunity benefits on a much deeper level. Making this treatment a part of your wellness regimen or seeking relief from a chronic condition can make lymphatic Drainage Massage a valuable complement to your traditional healthcare.

CHAPTER THREE

HEALTH BENEFITS OF LYMPHATIC DRAINAGE MASSAGE

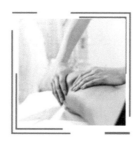

In the realm of holistic health practices, Lymphatic Drainage Massage has garnered increasing attention for its profound, positive impact on people's health. In the last chapter, we introduced the science of Lymphatic Drainage Massage, its effects on the internal systems, and how to visually identify when therapy is needed.

Now, we will discuss the health benefits and specific conditions that improve with this therapy. Lymphatic Drainage Massage can also be integrated with holistic treatments such as acupuncture, chiropractic care, and herbal medicine, along with traditional healthcare, to enhance overall health.

IMMUNE HEALTH

Lymphatic Drainage Massage boosts our immune system by improving lymphatic circulation, which helps spread immune cells across the body. When lymph flow improves, our bodies can fight infections more effectively. For instance, if someone catches a cold, they may recover faster and with fewer symptoms. Because transporting white blood cells is critical in battling infections, it is crucial for this to happen during cold and flu season or when infections are more common. Chronic diseases like recurrent ear or respiratory ailments and allergic reactions benefit from regularly practicing Lymphatic Drainage Massage. This holistic approach not only helps immunity but also improves overall health.

People with weak immune systems, like those going through cancer treatment or living with long-term health problems, can find relief. Patients undergoing chemotherapy might also feel that Lymphatic Drainage Massage helps ease their physical pain and promotes relaxation.

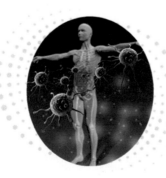

Illustration of immunity against diseases

It is recommended to Combine Lymphatic Drainage Massage with healthy habits such as staying hydrated, eating a balanced diet with plenty of vitamins and minerals, and being physically active. Drinking enough water is particularly important because it helps thin out the lymphatic fluid, making it easier for the system to work. Remember, when we boost the lymph flow and clean the system, we increase overall immune health.

DETOXIFICATION

Toxins can accumulate due to environmental factors, diet, and lifestyle choices. When these harmful substances build up, they can impair the immune system, making it harder for our bodies to fight off illnesses. The gentle techniques used in Lymphatic Drainage Massage move stagnated lymph fluid, carrying toxins away from the tissues to the bloodstream for excretion.

During times of illness, our bodies can build up toxins from medicines, antibiotics, and even chemotherapy. These toxins can settle in different body tissues. Lymphatic Drainage Massage aids in the removal of these excess toxins, leading to faster healing, less brain fog, and a healthier body.

Detoxification can also benefit smokers by lessening cravings and improving mood, making it easier to quit the habit. By ridding the body of toxins, the recovery can make people feel lighter and better. Clean blood and bodily fluids bring more nutrients and oxygen to the cells. Increased energy and clearer thinking are some of these benefits.

STRESS / RELAXATION

Chronic stress can harm the lymphatic system and overall health. Finding time to relax can reduce stress. Relaxation methods like deep breathing, meditation, or taking short breaks can significantly help as well. Additionally, gentle Lymphatic Drainage Massages or calm yoga can relieve tension and keep the lymphatic system running smoothly.

Stress affects many areas of our health, especially with various diseases. Whether it's a short-term or long-term issue, stress strongly impacts the body. It can make discomfort worse and affect conditions like swelling. When stressed, the body may struggle to manage fluid levels. Relaxation is crucial for our body's best performance. Rest allows time for recovery and healing. During rest, our bodies can work on detoxifying and healing pain. People may notice more aches or digestive problems when stressed for long periods. Having a routine that includes relaxation can make a big difference. This could be as easy as setting aside time daily to unwind. Activities like reading, taking a warm bath, doing breathing exercises, or lymphatic massages can positively affect the nervous system lowering stress levels and making people feel calmer.

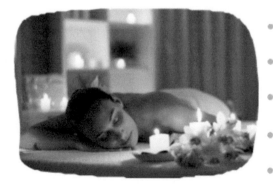

When we handle stress well, we usually feel happier and more balanced. Many people have more significant cognitive thinking and are more and more satisfied after a good lymphatic drainage session or similar relaxation methods. Taking time each day to relax reduces stress and helps create a positive mindset. Journaling, listening to soothing music, or walking in nature can help mental balance. Remember that relaxation can be simple; it may be as easy as enjoying a cup of tea quietly or talking with a friend.

When you practice relaxation techniques, you may find managing chronic pain better. Over time, having fewer flare-ups can lessen the need for medications, giving you more control and independence. Creating a personal relaxation space in your room, with soft cushions and calming decorations, can also help. This area should be inviting and free from distractions. Consider adding things like candles, soothing sounds, or plants. Making this small investment in your space can encourage you to take time to relax.

As you manage stress, you must check in with yourself regularly. Being aware of your feelings helps you notice patterns and triggers more easily. Ask yourself, "How am I feeling right now?" or "What can I do today to take care of myself?" Awareness of your emotions helps you manage stress before it gets too much. Over time, this will help you develop healthier habits and feel more at peace.

SKIN HEALTH

Lymphatic Drainage Massage is a necessary process that can help improve the look and health of your skin. It can also improve skin conditions like acne, eczema, and psoriasis. These conditions often involve inflammation, which can get worse if not treated. The lymphatic system location is just beneath the skin's surface and is crucial for removing waste and extracellular fluid from the tissues. If the lymph is not flowing correctly, it can cause a buildup of toxins and fluid. This can lead to a dull complexion and puffiness. To avoid these issues, it's essential to assist the lymphatic system. This can be achieved with Lymphatic Drainage Massages and some lifestyle changes.

The lymphatic techniques not only reduces inflammation, but also swelling and bloating. When the lymphatic system is working well, increased blood flow brings oxygen and nutrients to the skin cells. This is necessary for healthy skin. Therefore, when blood reaches the cells efficiently, your skin gets the nutrients it needs to function well and look good. A healthy diet, quality skincare products, regular exercise, drinking enough water, and caring for your skin can enhance your health and appearance.

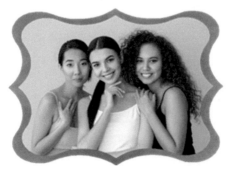

PAIN RELIEF

For individuals suffering from chronic pain conditions, we know from Chapter 1 that a healthy lymph flow impacts muscles, venous flow, and nerve tissues. Lymphatic Drainage Massage lessens restriction, improves joint mobility, reduces inflammation, and improves circulation. Therapists can positively impact diseases that cause inflammation, such as arthritis, fibromyalgia, etc., reduce pain, and can also be used as pain management.

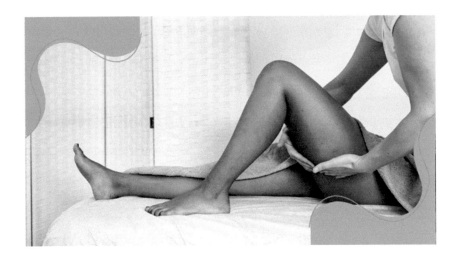

SWELLING / EDEMA

Two conditions that cause chronic swelling/edema are lymphedema and lipedema. Lymphedema involves the accumulation of fluid, whereas lipedema consists of the accumulation of fat tissue. A few other common health conditions, such as pregnancy, diabetes, gut health, weight loss, and post-surgery, can cause severe or chronic swelling. These conditions present visually and indicate that Lymphatic Drainage Massage would be beneficial by improving lymph flow, thereby reducing fluid retention and discomfort.

1. **Lymphedema:** Lymphedema is a severe, chronic medical condition characterized by the accumulation of lymph fluid in the tissues leading to swelling, typically in the arms, hips, or legs. It's an edema that is the result of impaired removal of lymph. This occurs when the lymphatic system is damaged or blocked, preventing the proper drainage of lymph fluid. The swelling can lead to discomfort, limited mobility, skin changes, and an increased risk of infections. The therapist can decrease the fluid from outside the lymph system to create a fluid balance that needs to be regularly maintained. With regular therapy, clients may be able to experience less pain, tension, and joint stress.

There are various reasons that Lymphedema can occur. The primary reason is due to a congenital disorder with which the person is born.

The secondary reason is due to an injury or incident that disrupts the lymphatic system.

Primary Cause of Lymphedema - congenital origin (birth) Secondary Causes of Lymphedema - origins of various causes:

- surgeries and biopsies
- radiation therapy
- burns and trauma
- parasites, infections, etc.
- a chronic venous condition
- cancers (lymphoma, breast, pelvic, prostate, etc.)

2. Lipedema: Lipedema is a chronic disorder of the adipose (fat) tissue characterized by the symmetrical accumulation of fat in the legs, hips, and sometimes the arms. This condition is a common but under-recognized disorder predominantly affecting women. It is often mistaken for simple obesity or lymphedema. Lipedema may cause pain, swelling, and easy bruising, sometimes accompanied by an unusual texture within the fat tissue that can feel like rice, peas, or walnuts beneath the skin's surface.

Lipedema pain can range from none to severe, the frequency may be constant, it may come and go, or it may only present when manipulated. The symptoms, as well as the stress of this condition, can lead to physical and emotional distress, fatigue, and muscle pain. Unlike Lymphedema, Lipedema is not caused by a blockage in the lymphatic system but is believed to have a genetic and hormonal basis. There are many ways a therapist can help with this condition, such as using Lymphatic Drainage Massage to release toxins and clear the tissue, as well as from a cellulite treatment standpoint. Performing a fascia release technique, which can allow the tissue to have more freedom, can decrease pain in muscles and joints, allowing more muscle fiber movement. A treatment called SculptICE or Cryo- therapy can decrease fat tissue and bring the area treated a slimmer look, allowing the client to have more confidence. Another manual technique called skin rolling will help with collagen and elastin production for fuller and smoother skin texture. All of these treatments will address fat tissue, tightness, pain, and skin elasticity while decreasing the size of the limb.

Some key differences between the two conditions are:

Tissue Involved: Lymphedema involves lymph fluid accumulation in tissues, leading to swelling. Lipedema involves an abnormal accumulation of fat cells.

Location of Swelling: Lymphedema typically affects one limb or part of a limb, whereas Lipedema usually affects both legs symmetrically and may also involve the arms.

Symptoms: Lymphedema symptoms include swelling, skin changes, and a higher risk of infection. Lipedema symptoms include painful fat deposits, easy bruising, and tenderness.

Both conditions can significantly impact quality of life and require different management and treatment approaches. Proper diagnosis by a healthcare professional is essential for effective treatment and management. Dealing with Lymphedema and Lipedema can be a lonely, frustrating journey.

Some primary treatment goals are to:

- Manage Inflammation

- Improve Lymphatic Flow

- Reduce Fibrosis

- Manage Pain

- Decrease Adipose Tissue

- Promote Healthy lifestyle

- Prioritize Emotional/Mental Health

While there is currently no cure, having a lymphatic massage routine and self-care home regimen is effective at managing symptoms and improving the quality of life for patients. While surgery such as liposuction can be valuable for some lipedema patients to improve mobility and visual appearance, it is still not a cure for the condition.

When it comes to Lymphedema, there are specific stages to the disorder; thus, there are also correlating levels of therapist certification for treatments. I have currently worked with clients in the early stages of it. Manual treatment and the Endosphere device have given my clients great benefits and remarkable results in decreasing swelling and maintaining Lymphedema.

I have treated clients with lipedema by dry brushing, a skin rolling technique, Lymphatic Drainage Massage, and treatments that decrease fat cells. These techniques allow the fascia to be loosened and fluids to be removed from the fat cells.

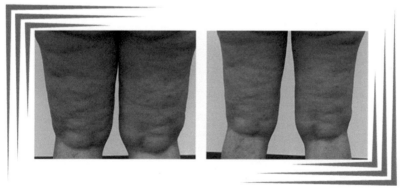

*Actual Lipedema Client after six
Lymphatic Drainage Therapies.*

Illustration of Lymphedema vs Lipedema

LYMPHEDEMA

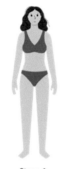 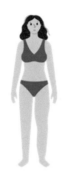 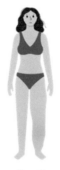 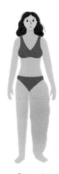

Stage 1
Abnormal flow in the lymphatic system.
No symptoms

Stage 2
Accumulation of fluid with swelling.
Pressing on the area may leave a dent

Stage 3
Changes in the skin
with scarring and thickening

Stage 4
Large deformed limb,
extensive scarring

LIPEDEMA

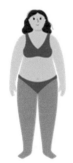 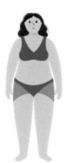 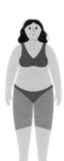 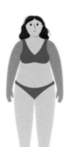 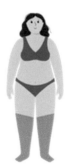

3. Pregnancy: Pregnancy often leads to increased fluid retention, particularly in the legs, ankles, and feet. This condition, known as edema, results in swelling and discomfort for the pregnant mother. As the baby grows in the womb, the added pressure on the veins constricts the venous flow. Added to this are hormonal fluctuations that also increase pressure on blood vessels, leading to fluid retention.

As the pregnancy continues to progress, the mother may begin to experience aches and pains, particularly in the lower back, hips, and legs. These discomforts can intensify due to the added weight of the growing baby, coupled with fluid retention. Regular massages can significantly alleviate these issues by reducing inflammation and enhancing tissue mobility. The improved circulation also helps mitigate the severity of varicose veins, which can develop due to the increased pressure. Targeted massages help maintain muscle strength and flexibility, preparing the mother for childbirth and contributing to a more favorable birthing experience.

Lymphatic Drainage Massage serves as an effective remedy for fluid retention. Think of it as facilitating the body's natural process to eliminate excess fluid and waste. As Lymphatic Drainage Massage improves the circulation of lymph and blood, crucial nutrients and oxygen are delivered to both mother and baby. Thus, this type of massage not only alleviates discomfort, but also promotes the health of the unborn child.

When searching for a therapist, it's crucial to select someone experienced in prenatal care. This expert should be well-versed in prenatal massage techniques and lymphatic drainage. They must have the skills and knowledge to provide safe treatments tailored to a woman's specific needs during pregnancy. Their understanding of the physiological changes in a woman's body during pregnancy allows them to offer safe, effective treatments. Inquiring about the therapist's training and experience can help the mother find someone who offers effective and reassuring care.

While the benefits of Lymphatic Drainage Massage during pregnancy are evident, it's vital to engage in open discussions with healthcare providers before beginning any new treatment. Gaining approval from a physician or qualified practitioner ensures that therapy, including Lymphatic Drainage Massage, aligns with each pregnant woman's unique health status.

In conjunction with professional massages, pregnant women can explore self-care techniques and exercises at home. Regular movement is vital in maintaining circulation, helping to combat the heaviness and discomfort that many women experience.

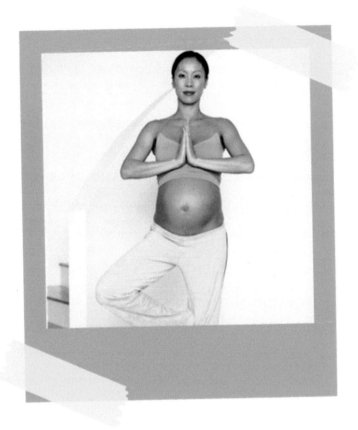

Engaging in gentle stretching or light walking helps boost circulation and reduce swelling. Staying hydrated is essential for flushing out excess sodium and minimizing fluid retention. Consuming a balanced diet filled with fruits, vegetables, and lean proteins supports overall health during pregnancy. Moreover, elevating the legs during rest can significantly alleviate swelling. Placing pillows under the legs or feet while lying down promotes better blood flow and reduces fluid build-up. This simple adjustment can yield noticeable comfort after a tiring day.

2. Diabetes: Massage can help those with diabetes by reducing swelling and moving lymph fluid. People with diabetes commonly experience foot and leg swelling and skin breakdown, leading to ulcers, kidney issues, and neuropathy in their hands or feet, causing numbness and pain. Relieving fluid pressure can reduce swelling and tightness, making limbs feel lighter and more comfortable. This also lowers the risk of skin issues, infections, and kidney complications while improving nerve function and reducing numbness and pain.

Thanks to the relaxation gained from Lymphatic Drainage Massage, sleep quality can also improve. Many people with diabetes struggle with sleep because of medications, discomfort, or anxiety. By making massage a calming routine, individuals may find it easier to have deeper, more restful sleep, helping their bodies recover.

Good sleep and lowering hormone levels are essential for managing diabetes because controlling blood sugar helps maintain energy. People with diabetes can experience frustration trying to balance their glucose and their fluid retention. By becoming more relaxed through massage and meditation, they can experience a reduction in mental stress and anxiety. Thus, lowering stress hormones is crucial because it assists with blood sugar control.

Many patients notice improvement, making it easier to stay more active and keep their blood sugar levels steady. Clarity is another benefit of relaxation, making it easier to make better food choices and stick to exercises. Last, Lymphatic Drainage Massage can also provide emotional support; many people with diabetes feel lonely. Having a therapist who understands diabetes and offers a range of tips and lifestyle suggestions can boost confidence.

5. Gut Health and Weight Loss: The human body is an intricate system where everything is interconnected. The lymphatic system plays a pivotal role, particularly in gut health and weight management. Lymphatic Drainage Massage can be a powerful tool for enhancing gut function and supporting weight loss.

Unlike the cardiovascular system, which uses the heart to pump blood, the lymphatic system relies on muscle movement and deep breathing to circulate lymph fluid throughout the body.

The lymphatic system in our gut is primarily made up of lymphatic vessels and structures known as Peyer's patches, clusters of lymphoid tissue located in the small intestine. These lymphoid tissues are essential for filtering and responding to pathogens, and they also play a role in the absorption of dietary fats and fat-soluble vitamins through specialized lymphatic vessels called lacteals.

The Gut-Lymph connection profoundly impacts our health and is often called the body's "second brain." It houses trillions of microorganisms that influence everything from digestion to mood. Intimately connected, our gut and the lymphatic system tissue predominately reside in our abdominal region. This connection plays a vital role in our immune function and the absorption of nutrients,

If our lymphatic system functions appropriately, lymph fluid circulates efficiently, picking up waste products, toxins, and excess fluid from tissues. It then transports them to lymph nodes for filtration, which helps to keep our body's internal environment clean and balanced. This is particularly important because of the vast array of nutrients, waste products, and potentially harmful substances.

When the lymphatic system is sluggish or congested, it can lead to poor gut health and stagnation in the gut, which leads to symptoms like bloating, constipation, and inflammation. A well-functioning lymphatic system supports the gut by removing toxins and reducing inflammation, which in turn can improve digestion and nutrient absorption. Lymphatic sluggishness or congestion can occur due to a variety of factors. Some common causes include:

- Poor Diet: A diet high in sugar, processed foods, and unhealthy fats can lead to the buildup of toxins and inflammation in the gut. This affects digestion and places additional stress on the lymphatic system, leading to congestion.

- Lack of Physical Activity: Movement is essential for lymphatic circulation since the lymphatic system does not have a central pump like the heart. A sedentary lifestyle can slow lymph flow, causing fluid retention and congestion.

- Chronic: Stress profoundly impacts the body's systems, including the lymphatic system. Chronic stress can lead to inflammation, contributing to lymphatic congestion and sluggishness that can disrupt the gut.

- Dehydration: Proper hydration is crucial for maintaining the viscosity and flow of lymph fluid. Without adequate water intake, lymph fluid can become thick and slow-moving, leading to congestion.

- Digestive Disorders: Conditions like irritable bowel syndrome (IBS), leaky gut syndrome, and chronic constipation can disrupt the balance of the gut microbiome and increase inflammation, which can, in turn, affect lymphatic function within the gut.

- Toxin Overload: Exposure to environmental toxins, heavy metals, and chemicals can burden the lymphatic system, leading to congestion as the system struggles to filter out these harmful substances.

Weight loss is often a complex and multifaceted journey involving diet, exercise, and lifestyle changes. However, lymphatic drainage massage can support weight loss by helping the body efficiently eliminate waste and toxins, supporting metabolic processes, and improving energy levels.

Lymphatic Drainage Massage aids in weight loss, leading to a slimmer appearance and reduced body weight. It can help regulate appetite, reduce cravings, improve the absorption of nutrients, support the body's natural detoxification processes, and improve metabolism, all of which are important for sustainable weight loss. This can also make it easier to maintain an active lifestyle.

6. Post Surgery: Lymphatic Drainage Massage is beneficial in the recovery process following surgery as it aids in reducing swelling, minimizing scar tissue formation, and accelerating the healing process. Surgical procedures can cause trauma to the body, and because of this trauma, the lymphatic system can become sluggish, leading to fluid retention and increased inflammation in the surgical area. Lymphatic Drainage Massage helps to minimize or alleviate these issues by enhancing circulation, reducing discomfort, and promoting a smoother recovery.

It is particularly recommended for surgeries like cesarian /abdominal procedures, which can impact the small intestines, cosmetic procedures, orthopedic surgeries, where a lot of scraping can cause congestion and mobility restrictions, transplants, and lymph node removals, where managing swelling and optimizing healing is crucial. Please consult your healthcare provider to ensure this massage therapy is appropriate for your post-surgical needs.

7. Inflammatory conditions: Lymphatic drainage massage can benefit those with inflammatory conditions—the buildup of toxins and fluids in tissues, which the lymphatic system is designed to remove. This specialized massage technique can help decrease inflammation, relieve pain, and promote healing by gently stimulating lymph flow. Enhanced lymphatic function also boosts immune response, allowing the body to process and eliminate toxins and pathogens more efficiently. For individuals with chronic inflammation, regular Lymphatic Drainage Massage can effectively manage symptoms and support overall tissue health.

Some inflammatory conditions where Lymphatic Drainage Massage is helpful:

- Chronic Fatigue Syndrome (CFS).
- Arthritis
- Fibromyalgia
- Sinusitis
- Migraines and Chronic Headaches
- Crohn's
- H. Pylori
- Lupus
- Multiple SclerOsis

HEALTH CONTRAINDICATIONS

Individuals and Therapists must use common sense. If you have any doubts or are unsure about your health condition, always seek the guidance of your physician. Even though there are many health benefits to having Lymphatic Drainage Massage, there are also contraindications. Here is a list of various conditions:

Acute Illnesses or Infections (with)

- Fever
- Bacterial Infections
- Influenza
- Inflammation accompanied by a fever
  (can start if the fever has been broken for 24-72 hours)
- Cellulitis (stop treatment for 5-8 days)

Serious Circulatory and Cardiac Problems

Lymphatic Drainage Massage is helpful in most instances except those listed below, which are contraindicated:

- Thrombosis (DO NOT RISK due to possible embolism)
- Aortic Aneurysm
- Venous (vein obstruction)
- Brachiocephalic (upper arm) obstruction
- Acute Angina (chest area)
- Coronary Thrombosis (heart attack)
- Congestive Heart Failure (cardiac insufficiency) because it increases the cardiac load

Hemorrhage (internal bleeding)

- This is contraindicated for internal bleeding issues.

Acute Anuresis

- This is contraindicated if you are having issues with urinating.

Active Cancer (undiagnosed lump)

- This is contraindicated unless you work with a provider who has approved your treatment.

Edema /Lymphedema

- This is contraindicated with severe edema of the heart, kidney, or liver.

- Chronic or later stages of Lymphedema should be done ONLY by a trained nurse, physical therapist, or massage therapist with extensive training. MAKE SURE TO ASK THE LEVEL OF EXPERTISE.

Hyper- and Hypo- Thyroid

- This is contraindicated due to the possibility of disrupting the blood- hormone ratio.

Burns and Fresh Scars

- This is contraindicated unless ordered by a physician or dermatologist.

Menstruation / Gynecological Infections

- This is contraindicated during the menstrual cycle and/or heavy bleeding.

- Avoid deep lymphatic drainage with a cyst, an IUD, or an infection.

Medications

- This is contraindicated during Chemotherapy and with Anesthetic drugs, which may circulate or be metabolized. Physicians may have to adjust medications.

As a rule of thumb, Lymphatic Drainage Massage must be avoided during all crisis periods and should never cause pain.

CHAPTER FOUR

LYMPHATIC DEVICES, SELECTING A THERAPIST, AND SELF-CARE TECHNIQUES

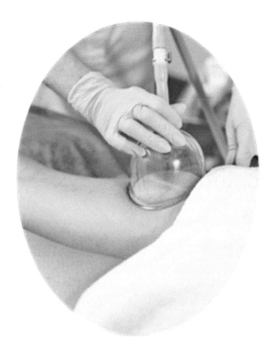

We now have newer technology and electronic devices that complement the Lymphatic Drainage Massage experience. Previously, we discussed the manual massage experience. Now we will dive into the mechanical options available which allow the therapist to provide clients with a different modality. A few of these devices are Cupping/MediCupping, Pressotherapy, Endermologie, and Endosphere therapies.

Cupping/ MediCupping:

One remarkable lymphatic method is Medicupping, which creates a "separation" effect when a vacuum is used. This technique employs a distinct negative pressure that can only be achieved with this vacuum device. The cups glide over the skin using various motions such as gliding, shaking, twisting, and rotating while the cup is being gently lifted by the machine. This process promotes water absorption and enhances blood circulation, facilitating the nourishment and hydration of tissues. This is particularly beneficial before and after surgical procedures. It is clear that by separating congested tissue and soft tissue, adherence can enhance functionality and stimulate improvements in numerous health conditions.

Lymphatic Devices Cont.

Treatments can be performed at any time, either directly on bare skin or with a lubricant for optimal movement. After just a few sessions, tissues can successfully absorb water and nutrients, achieving a healthy, moist state. This rehydration allows for the removal of waste products that could lead to allergies, inflammation, or sensitivities. Furthermore, this technique supports vascular health and promotes collagen synthesis, which aids in firming lax tissue. Even when addressing deep scars, adhesions, fibrous tissue, or fascia, this innovative "lifting without force" approach recalls the body's memory while providing a comfortable, rapid therapeutic experience.

Endermologie

A cutting-edge procedure known as Endermologie® was developed to effectively diminish stubborn fat deposits and enhance skin texture by reducing the visibility of cellulite without the need for invasive surgery. Its capability to stimulate fluid movement not only aids in stretching connective tissue but also revitalizes skin health and softens scar tissue. This innovative machine can also alleviate pain and muscle spasms, promote collagen production, reduce fine lines and wrinkles, and firm slightly sagging skin, all while enhancing both blood and lymphatic circulation.

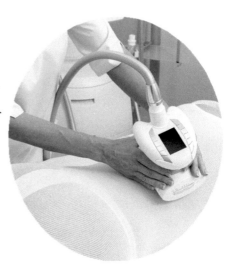

This treatment can be performed 1-2 times a week, bi-weekly, monthly, or when needed for regular maintenance, and is typically sold in packages. When receiving treatments, the client must wear a full-body stocking suit, as this procedure is not performed on bare skin.

Pressotherapy

Pressotherapy is a medical and cosmetic treatment that uses air pressure to stimulate the lymphatic system, improve circulation, and reduce swelling. This noninvasive procedure is often used to improve venous circulation, treat conditions like Lymphedema, and promote overall lymphatic health.

Here's how Pressotherapy operates: Pressotherapy utilizes specialized garments consisting of a fitted jacket or pants with numerous air chambers. These garments are strategically positioned on targeted areas of the body. The air chambers deliver pressure to regions such as the legs, arms, or abdomen through inflating and deflating in a systematic, sequential fashion. This action simulates natural muscle contractions during physical activity, facilitating lymphatic drainage and enhancing blood circulation. Pressure levels can be customized to meet the individual's requirements and the conditions being addressed.

A healthcare professional will assess the patient's condition and determine the appropriate settings for the Pressotherapy session. A typical Pressotherapy session lasts between 30 to 45 minutes.

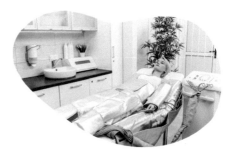

Micro-Vibration Therapy

Micro-vibration therapy is one of the latest cutting-edge treatments that uses a rolling device comprised of over 50 soft silicone spheres. Due to the gentle vibrations, a therapist can work on slow lymphatic flow, stagnant fluids, and tight fascia that have trapped fatty tissue causing the appearance of cellulite. Restoring circulation reduces puffiness and improves the appearance of stretch marks, scars, and wrinkles, toning and firming the tissues and giving a more youthful appearance. The treatment is non-invasive, making it safe and effective.

This treatment can be performed weekly, bi-weekly, monthly, or when needed for regular maintenance and is typically sold in packages.

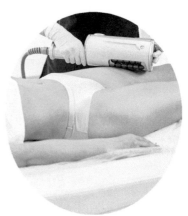

Depending on your therapist, all of these devices and many more may be used in conjunction with lymphatic drainage techniques. Whether you choose a manual technique, a device, or a combination of both, you now have a wealth of knowledge and the tools you need to Flow and thrive to the fullest.

Lymphatic Therapist

Professional lymphatic drainage requires finding a certified therapist who specializes in this field. Look for a practitioner who has undergone comprehensive training in lymphatic drainage techniques, such as those developed by Vodder or Chickley. Verify that the therapist's certification is not just a brief course but is quality training. A qualified therapist should be able to articulate a session structure, demonstrate an understanding of your specific condition, and comprehend the objectives you wish to achieve. Additionally, they should clearly grasp the differences between lymphatic fluid and fat and manage both.

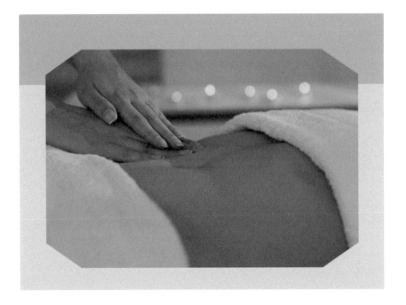

Lymphatic Drainage Self-Care

Self-care is about honoring your needs and nurturing your well-being, preparing for your mind to receive and your body to release. It's a pause, a breath, and a focus on feeling refreshed and fulfilled. Embrace this time to pamper yourself and remember that caring for your mind, body, and spirit is not just a luxury—it's essential for a balanced and healthy life.

We created an in-home, self-care experience for you to enjoy. Please feel free to use the following QR codes to relax and enhance your regimen. Choose from a Spa or Soulful experience.

Soul Relaxing

Spa Melodies

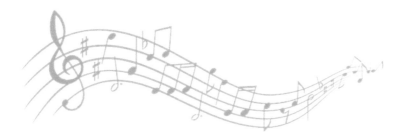

Simple lymphatic drainage techniques are meant for individuals to practice at home. To effectively learn these techniques, you can seek instruction from a qualified therapist who can guide you through the right methods. Understanding which areas to target, the appropriate pressure to apply, and the correct flow direction is crucial.

Establishing a self-care regimen for lymphatic drainage can enhance your lymphatic system's function and contribute to your health and wellness. Next are simple routines designed to help you embark on your health journey in the comfort of your home.

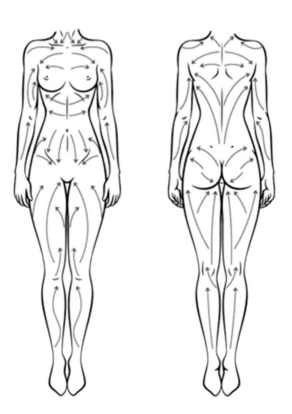

Illustration of Lymphatic Drainage Flow

DAILY ROUTINE

MORNING:

Hydrate:

- Drink a glass of warm water with lemon. This helps kickstart your metabolism and promotes lymphatic flow.

Dry Brushing:

- Brush with a natural bristle brush. Brush with small, quick strokes toward the lymph nodes, working your way to stoke up longer the entire limb and & abdomen toward the heart.

Technique:

- Start clearing the lymph nodes with rhythmic pulsing at your collarbone. Continue the rhythmic pulsing at the armpits, infolds of the arms, lower abdomen, upper inner thighs, and behind the knees and ankles. Then, begin brushing at your feet, moving toward your heart. Use a long, sweeping motion, brushing each area of your body, including your legs, arms, back, and torso.

Duration:

- Spend about 5-10 minutes on this routine.

Exercises:

- Stretch, rebound, walk briefly, or do gentle yoga.

THROUGHOUT THE DAY

Stay Hydrated:

- Drink 8-10 glasses of water throughout the day and stay hydrated.

- Eat foods containing water, such as cucumbers, watermelon, and celery, to help maintain lymph fluid balance and support detoxification.

Move Regularly:

- Stretch every hour and take short breaks.

- Walk for exercise and do light stretching to prevent stagnation and support lymph flow.

EVENING

- Start with rhythmic pulsing of the lymph nodes at your collarbone. Then, begin to brush at your feet, moving toward your heart. Use a long, sweeping motion, brushing each area of your body, including your legs, arms, back, and torso.

Techniques: (Massage with your hands or a gentle massager)

- **Massage Face and Head:** Glide your fingers lightly in a circular or lifting motion, starting from the center of your face and moving outward.

- **Massage Arms:** Sweep with your fingertips moving towards the shoulders with gentle, brushing strokes.

- **Massage Legs:** Stroke with full hands in upward stroking movements starting at the feet and moving toward the hips. Then, elevate your legs for up to fifteen minutes.

- **Massage Abdomen:** Glide your palms, hand over hand, in a circular, clockwise motion.

- Spend 15-20 minutes with this routine.

Relaxation and Deep Breathing:

- Practice deep belly breathing exercises or meditation.

- Spend 10-15 minutes.

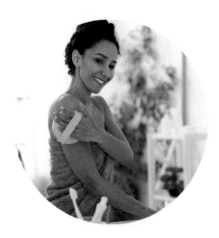

Epsom Salt Bath

Ingredients:

- Pour two cups of Epsom salts into a warm bath to promote relaxation and detoxification. The magnesium in the salts rejuvenates muscles and promotes relaxation.

Duration:

- Soak for 20-30 minutes.

Exercise:

- Walk briskly, swim, or rebound. Aerobic workouts increase circulation and flow.

Duration:

- Spend 30-45 minutes per session.

Frequency:

- Incorporate this routine at least three times a week.

Healthy Eating

Diet:

- Eat foods like fruits, vegetables, lean proteins, and healthy fats.

Hydration:

- Consume hydrating foods such as cucumbers, watermelon, leafy greens, and water.

MONTHLY ROUTINE

Professional Lymphatic Drainage Massage

Frequency:

- Schedule with a therapist monthly or as recommended to provide a deeper level of lymphatic drainage and to address any specific concerns.

ADDITIONAL TIPS

Rest:

- Aim for 7-8 hours of quality sleep nightly.

Manage Stress:

- Practice stress-reducing activities such as meditation, deep breathing, and hobbies you enjoy.

Reduce Toxins:

- Reduce toxin exposure. Limit alcohol, caffeine, and processed foods.

Clothing:

- Wear loose, comfortable clothing to avoid restricting lymphatic flow.

CONCLUSION

Incorporating self-care practices into daily, weekly, and monthly routines supports your lymphatic system, enhances your immune function, and promotes a healthy lifestyle. Remember to listen to your body and adjust the protocol as needed. Consult with a healthcare professional if you have any medical conditions or concerns.

SOURCES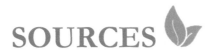

Kellogg, John Harvey. *The Art of Massage*, Modern Medicine
Publishing, 1929.

Adair, TH, Guyton. *Experimental Biology of the Lymphatic
Circulation*, Elsevier, 1985.

Chickley, Bruno. Upledger Foundation Course, *Lymphatic Pathways:
Anatomical Integrity,* 2007.

Wiltsie, Charles W. III, and Katherine M. *Lypossage, 12th Edition.*
Self Published, 2020.

Warner, Ruth. *A Massage Therapist Guide to Pathology, 2nd Edition,*
Lippincott Williams & Wilkins, 2002.

Salvo, Susan G. *Massage Therapy Principles and Practice, 5th Edition,*
Elsevier Publishing, 2016.

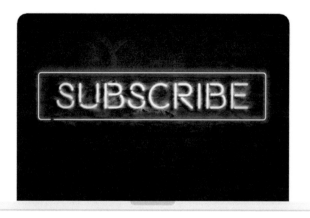

YouTube - Podcast Coming Soon!

Coming soon! Please subscribe to our *Waze2Wellness* YouTube channel and Podcast. Join us weekly as we do a dive deep into alternative ways to health, wellness, and natural healing practices from a therapeutic standpoint of massage, acupuncture, herbal, and functional medicine. Each episode features interviews with health professionals and real clients providing insightful discussions along with practical tips to help you integrate these therapies into your daily life. Whether you're a wellness enthusiast or just curious about alternative healing, *Waze2Wellness* offers valuable information and inspiration to guide you on your journey to a healthier, balanced, and more vibrant life.

YT: @waze2wellness

email: waze2wellness@gmail.com

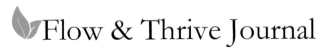Flow & Thrive Journal

Date
_____

I am capable, strong, and ready to take on the day.
Today, I choose joy, peace, and positivity in all I do.
_____

Today, I woke up and I appreciate it because:
_____
_____
_____
_____

Today, my health gratitude is:
_____
_____
_____
_____

Today, I discovered this about my health and/or self-care:
_____
_____
_____
_____

Today, was not a good day, and this is how I handled it:
_____
_____
_____
_____

FLOW & THRIVE
WEEKLY CHECKLIST

Journaling healthcare is a loving commitment to oneself.
How did you cherish yourself this week?

( ) Woke up restful most days ( ) Meet daily water intake

( ) Went for short walk ( ) Listen to favorite music

( ) Went for a long walk ( ) Spent time with a loved one

( ) Practice mindful meditation ( ) Pampered yourself

( ) Engaged in positive thinking ( ) Read for pleasure

( ) Stretching / Yoga ( ) Cooked a nourishing meal

( ) Worked out 3x or more ( ) Practice gratitude

Add any additional self cherishes or health changes.

_____

_____

_____

_____

_____

_____

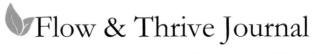Flow & Thrive Journal

Date
_____

I am capable, strong, and ready to take on the day.
Today, I choose joy, peace, and positivity in all I do.

_____

Today, I woke up and I appreciate it because:
_____
_____
_____
_____

Today, my health gratitude is:
_____
_____
_____
_____

Today, I discovered this about my health and/or self-care:
_____
_____
_____
_____

Today, was not a good day, and this is how I handled it:
_____
_____
_____
_____

FLOW & THRIVE
WEEKLY CHECKLIST

Journaling healthcare is a loving commitment to oneself.
How did you cherish yourself this week?

( ) Woke up restful most days   ( ) Meet daily water intake

( ) Went for short walk   ( ) Listen to favorite music

( ) Went for a long walk   ( ) Spent time with a loved one

( ) Practice mindful meditation   ( ) Pampered yourself

( ) Engaged in positive thinking   ( ) Read for pleasure

( ) Stretching / Yoga   ( ) Cooked a nourishing meal

( ) Worked out 3x or more   ( ) Practice gratitude

Add any additional self cherishes or health changes.

_____

_____

_____

_____

_____

_____

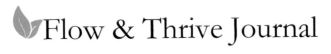Flow & Thrive Journal

Date
_____

I am capable, strong, and ready to take on the day.
Today, I choose joy, peace, and positivity in all I do.

_____

Today, I woke up and I appreciate it because:

_____
_____
_____
_____

Today, my health gratitude is:

_____
_____
_____
_____

Today, I discovered this about my health and/or self-care:

_____
_____
_____
_____

Today, was not a good day, and this is how I handled it:

_____
_____
_____
_____

FLOW & THRIVE
WEEKLY CHECKLIST

Journaling healthcare is a loving commitment to oneself.
How did you cherish yourself this week?

( ) Woke up restful most days   ( ) Meet daily water intake

( ) Went for short walk   ( ) Listen to favorite music

( ) Went for a long walk   ( ) Spent time with a loved one

( ) Practice mindful meditation ( ) Pampered yourself

( ) Engaged in positive thinking ( ) Read for pleasure

( ) Stretching / Yoga   ( ) Cooked a nourishing meal

( ) Worked out 3x or more   ( ) Practice gratitude

Add any additional self cherishes or health changes.

_____

_____

_____

_____

_____

_____

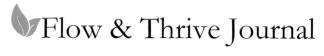# Flow & Thrive Journal

Date
_____

I am capable, strong, and ready to take on the day.
Today, I choose joy, peace, and positivity in all I do.
_____

Today, I woke up and I appreciate it because:
_____
_____
_____
_____

Today, my health gratitude is:
_____
_____
_____
_____

Today, I discovered this about my health and/or self-care:
_____
_____
_____
_____

Today, was not a good day, and this is how I handled it:
_____
_____
_____
_____

FLOW & THRIVE
WEEKLY CHECKLIST

Journaling healthcare is a loving commitment to oneself.
How did you cherish yourself this week?

( ) Woke up restful most days   ( ) Meet daily water intake

( ) Went for short walk   ( ) Listen to favorite music

( ) Went for a long walk   ( ) Spent time with a loved one

( ) Practice mindful meditation   ( ) Pampered yourself

( ) Engaged in positive thinking   ( ) Read for pleasure

( ) Stretching / Yoga   ( ) Cooked a nourishing meal

( ) Worked out 3x or more   ( ) Practice gratitude

Add any additional self cherishes or health changes.

_____

_____

_____

_____

_____

_____

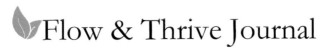Flow & Thrive Journal

Date

_____

I am capable, strong, and ready to take on the day.
Today, I choose joy, peace, and positivity in all I do.

_____

Today, I woke up and I appreciate it because:

_____

_____

_____

_____

Today, my health gratitude is:

_____

_____

_____

_____

Today, I discovered this about my health and/or self-care:

_____

_____

_____

_____

Today, was not a good day, and this is how I handled it:

_____

_____

_____

_____

FLOW & THRIVE
WEEKLY CHECKLIST

Journaling healthcare is a loving commitment to oneself.
How did you cherish yourself this week?

( ) Woke up restful most days   ( ) Meet daily water intake

( ) Went for short walk   ( ) Listen to favorite music

( ) Went for a long walk   ( ) Spent time with a loved one

( ) Practice mindful meditation   ( ) Pampered yourself

( ) Engaged in positive thinking   ( ) Read for pleasure

( ) Stretching / Yoga   ( ) Cooked a nourishing meal

( ) Worked out 3x or more   ( ) Practice gratitude

Add any additional self cherishes or health changes.

_____

_____

_____

_____

_____

_____

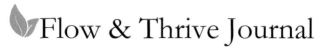# Flow & Thrive Journal

Date
_____

> I am capable, strong, and ready to take on the day.
> Today, I choose joy, peace, and positivity in all I do.

_____

Today, I woke up and I appreciate it because:

_____
_____
_____
_____

Today, my health gratitude is:

_____
_____
_____
_____

Today, I discovered this about my health and/or self-care:

_____
_____
_____
_____

Today, was not a good day, and this is how I handled it:

_____
_____
_____
_____

FLOW & THRIVE
WEEKLY CHECKLIST

Journaling healthcare is a loving commitment to oneself.
How did you cherish yourself this week?

( ) Woke up restful most days   ( ) Meet daily water intake

( ) Went for short walk   ( ) Listen to favorite music

( ) Went for a long walk   ( ) Spent time with a loved one

( ) Practice mindful meditation   ( ) Pampered yourself

( ) Engaged in positive thinking   ( ) Read for pleasure

( ) Stretching / Yoga   ( ) Cooked a nourishing meal

( ) Worked out 3x or more   ( ) Practice gratitude

Add any additional self cherishes or health changes.

_____

_____

_____

_____

_____

_____

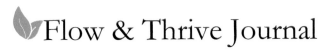Flow & Thrive Journal

Date

_____

I am capable, strong, and ready to take on the day.
Today, I choose joy, peace, and positivity in all I do.

_____

Today, I woke up and I appreciate it because:

_____
_____
_____
_____

Today, my health gratitude is:

_____
_____
_____
_____

Today, I discovered this about my health and/or self-care:

_____
_____
_____
_____

Today, was not a good day, and this is how I handled it:

_____
_____
_____

FLOW & THRIVE
WEEKLY CHECKLIST

Journaling healthcare is a loving commitment to oneself.
How did you cherish yourself this week?

( ) Woke up restful most days   ( ) Meet daily water intake

( ) Went for short walk   ( ) Listen to favorite music

( ) Went for a long walk   ( ) Spent time with a loved one

( ) Practice mindful meditation   ( ) Pampered yourself

( ) Engaged in positive thinking   ( ) Read for pleasure

( ) Stretching / Yoga   ( ) Cooked a nourishing meal

( ) Worked out 3x or more   ( ) Practice gratitude

Add any additional self cherishes or health changes.

_____

_____

_____

_____

_____

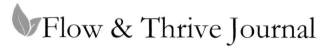Flow & Thrive Journal

Date
_____

> I am capable, strong, and ready to take on the day.
> Today, I choose joy, peace, and positivity in all I do.

_____

Today, I woke up and I appreciate it because:

_____
_____
_____
_____

Today, my health gratitude is:

_____
_____
_____
_____

Today, I discovered this about my health and/or self-care:

_____
_____
_____
_____

Today, was not a good day, and this is how I handled it:

_____
_____
_____
_____

FLOW & THRIVE
WEEKLY CHECKLIST

Journaling healthcare is a loving commitment to oneself.
How did you cherish yourself this week?

( ) Woke up restful most days   ( ) Meet daily water intake

( ) Went for short walk   ( ) Listen to favorite music

( ) Went for a long walk   ( ) Spent time with a loved one

( ) Practice mindful meditation   ( ) Pampered yourself

( ) Engaged in positive thinking   ( ) Read for pleasure

( ) Stretching / Yoga   ( ) Cooked a nourishing meal

( ) Worked out 3x or more   ( ) Practice gratitude

Add any additional self cherishes or health changes.

_____

_____

_____

_____

_____

_____

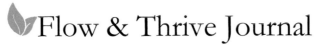# Flow & Thrive Journal

Date
_____

I am capable, strong, and ready to take on the day.
Today, I choose joy, peace, and positivity in all I do.
_____

Today, I woke up and I appreciate it because:
_____
_____
_____
_____

Today, my health gratitude is:
_____
_____
_____
_____

Today, I discovered this about my health and/or self-care:
_____
_____
_____
_____

Today, was not a good day, and this is how I handled it:
_____
_____
_____
_____

FLOW & THRIVE
WEEKLY CHECKLIST

Journaling healthcare is a loving commitment to oneself.
How did you cherish yourself this week?

( ) Woke up restful most days   ( ) Meet daily water intake

( ) Went for short walk   ( ) Listen to favorite music

( ) Went for a long walk   ( ) Spent time with a loved one

( ) Practice mindful meditation   ( ) Pampered yourself

( ) Engaged in positive thinking   ( ) Read for pleasure

( ) Stretching / Yoga   ( ) Cooked a nourishing meal

( ) Worked out 3x or more   ( ) Practice gratitude

Add any additional self cherishes or health changes.

_____

_____

_____

_____

_____

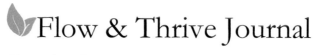Flow & Thrive Journal

Date
_____

I am capable, strong, and ready to take on the day.
Today, I choose joy, peace, and positivity in all I do.
_____

Today, I woke up and I appreciate it because:
_____
_____
_____
_____

Today, my health gratitude is:
_____
_____
_____
_____

Today, I discovered this about my health and/or self-care:
_____
_____
_____
_____

Today, was not a good day, and this is how I handled it:
_____
_____
_____
_____

FLOW & THRIVE
WEEKLY CHECKLIST

Journaling healthcare is a loving commitment to oneself.
How did you cherish yourself this week?

( ) Woke up restful most days   ( ) Meet daily water intake

( ) Went for short walk   ( ) Listen to favorite music

( ) Went for a long walk   ( ) Spent time with a loved one

( ) Practice mindful meditation   ( ) Pampered yourself

( ) Engaged in positive thinking   ( ) Read for pleasure

( ) Stretching / Yoga   ( ) Cooked a nourishing meal

( ) Worked out 3x or more   ( ) Practice gratitude

Add any additional self cherishes or health changes.

_____

_____

_____

_____

_____

_____

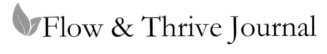Flow & Thrive Journal

Date
_____

I am capable, strong, and ready to take on the day.
Today, I choose joy, peace, and positivity in all I do.

_____

Today, I woke up and I appreciate it because:
_____
_____
_____
_____

Today, my health gratitude is:
_____
_____
_____
_____

Today, I discovered this about my health and/or self-care:
_____
_____
_____
_____

Today, was not a good day, and this is how I handled it:
_____
_____
_____
_____

FLOW & THRIVE
WEEKLY CHECKLIST

Journaling healthcare is a loving commitment to oneself.

How did you cherish yourself this week?

( ) Woke up restful most days   ( ) Meet daily water intake

( ) Went for short walk   ( ) Listen to favorite music

( ) Went for a long walk   ( ) Spent time with a loved one

( ) Practice mindful meditation   ( ) Pampered yourself

( ) Engaged in positive thinking   ( ) Read for pleasure

( ) Stretching / Yoga   ( ) Cooked a nourishing meal

( ) Worked out 3x or more   ( ) Practice gratitude

Add any additional self cherishes or health changes.

_____

_____

_____

_____

_____

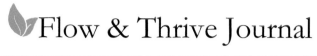# Flow & Thrive Journal

Date

_____

I am capable, strong, and ready to take on the day.
Today, I choose joy, peace, and positivity in all I do.

_____

Today, I woke up and I appreciate it because:

_____
_____
_____
_____

Today, my health gratitude is:

_____
_____
_____
_____

Today, I discovered this about my health and/or self-care:

_____
_____
_____
_____

Today, was not a good day, and this is how I handled it:

_____
_____
_____
_____

FLOW & THRIVE
WEEKLY CHECKLIST

Journaling healthcare is a loving commitment to oneself.

How did you cherish yourself this week?

( ) Woke up restful most days   ( ) Meet daily water intake

( ) Went for short walk   ( ) Listen to favorite music

( ) Went for a long walk   ( ) Spent time with a loved one

( ) Practice mindful meditation   ( ) Pampered yourself

( ) Engaged in positive thinking   ( ) Read for pleasure

( ) Stretching /Yoga   ( ) Cooked a nourishing meal

( ) Worked out 3x or more   ( ) Practice gratitude

Add any additional self cherishes or health changes.

_____

_____

_____

_____

_____

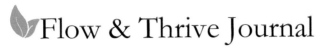
Flow & Thrive Journal

Date
_____

I am capable, strong, and ready to take on the day.
Today, I choose joy, peace, and positivity in all I do.
_____

Today, I woke up and I appreciate it because:
_____
_____
_____
_____

Today, my health gratitude is:
_____
_____
_____
_____

Today, I discovered this about my health and/or self-care:
_____
_____
_____
_____

Today, was not a good day, and this is how I handled it:
_____
_____
_____
_____

FLOW & THRIVE
WEEKLY CHECKLIST

Journaling healthcare is a loving commitment to oneself.

How did you cherish yourself this week?

( ) Woke up restful most days   ( ) Meet daily water intake

( ) Went for short walk   ( ) Listen to favorite music

( ) Went for a long walk   ( ) Spent time with a loved one

( ) Practice mindful meditation   ( ) Pampered yourself

( ) Engaged in positive thinking   ( ) Read for pleasure

( ) Stretching / Yoga   ( ) Cooked a nourishing meal

( ) Worked out 3x or more   ( ) Practice gratitude

Add any additional self cherishes or health changes.

_____

_____

_____

_____

_____

_____

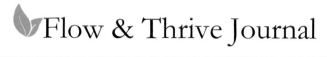Flow & Thrive Journal

Date

_____

I am capable, strong, and ready to take on the day.
Today, I choose joy, peace, and positivity in all I do.

_____

Today, I woke up and I appreciate it because:

_____
_____
_____
_____

Today, my health gratitude is:

_____
_____
_____
_____

Today, I discovered this about my health and/or self-care:

_____
_____
_____
_____

Today, was not a good day, and this is how I handled it:

_____
_____
_____
_____

FLOW & THRIVE
WEEKLY CHECKLIST

Journaling healthcare is a loving commitment to oneself.

How did you cherish yourself this week?

( ) Woke up restful most days   ( ) Meet daily water intake

( ) Went for short walk   ( ) Listen to favorite music

( ) Went for a long walk   ( ) Spent time with a loved one

( ) Practice mindful meditation   ( ) Pampered yourself

( ) Engaged in positive thinking   ( ) Read for pleasure

( ) Stretching / Yoga   ( ) Cooked a nourishing meal

( ) Worked out 3x or more   ( ) Practice gratitude

Add any additional self cherishes or health changes.

_____

_____

_____

_____

_____

_____

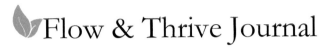Flow & Thrive Journal

Date

I am capable, strong, and ready to take on the day.
Today, I choose joy, peace, and positivity in all I do.

Today, I woke up and I appreciate it because:

_____

_____

_____

_____

Today, my health gratitude is:

_____

_____

_____

_____

Today, I discovered this about my health and/or self-care:

_____

_____

_____

_____

Today, was not a good day, and this is how I handled it:

_____

_____

_____

_____

FLOW & THRIVE
WEEKLY CHECKLIST

Journaling healthcare is a loving commitment to oneself.
How did you cherish yourself this week?

( ) Woke up restful most days   ( ) Meet daily water intake

( ) Went for short walk   ( ) Listen to favorite music

( ) Went for a long walk   ( ) Spent time with a loved one

( ) Practice mindful meditation   ( ) Pampered yourself

( ) Engaged in positive thinking   ( ) Read for pleasure

( ) Stretching / Yoga   ( ) Cooked a nourishing meal

( ) Worked out 3x or more   ( ) Practice gratitude

Add any additional self cherishes or health changes.

_____

_____

_____

_____

_____

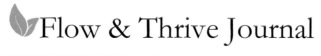Flow & Thrive Journal

Date
_____

I am capable, strong, and ready to take on the day.
Today, I choose joy, peace, and positivity in all I do.
_____

Today, I woke up and I appreciate it because:

_____
_____
_____
_____

Today, my health gratitude is:

_____
_____
_____
_____

Today, I discovered this about my health and/or self-care:

_____
_____
_____
_____

Today, was not a good day, and this is how I handled it:

_____
_____
_____
_____

FLOW & THRIVE
WEEKLY CHECKLIST

Journaling healthcare is a loving commitment to oneself.

How did you cherish yourself this week?

( ) Woke up restful most days   ( ) Meet daily water intake

( ) Went for short walk   ( ) Listen to favorite music

( ) Went for a long walk   ( ) Spent time with a loved one

( ) Practice mindful meditation   ( ) Pampered yourself

( ) Engaged in positive thinking   ( ) Read for pleasure

( ) Stretching / Yoga   ( ) Cooked a nourishing meal

( ) Worked out 3x or more   ( ) Practice gratitude

Add any additional self cherishes or health changes.

_____

_____

_____

_____

_____

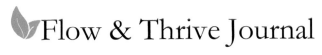Flow & Thrive Journal

Date
_____

I am capable, strong, and ready to take on the day.
Today, I choose joy, peace, and positivity in all I do.
_____

Today, I woke up and I appreciate it because:
_____
_____
_____
_____

Today, my health gratitude is:
_____
_____
_____
_____

Today, I discovered this about my health and/or self-care:
_____
_____
_____
_____

Today, was not a good day, and this is how I handled it:
_____
_____
_____
_____

FLOW & THRIVE
WEEKLY CHECKLIST

Journaling healthcare is a loving commitment to oneself.
How did you cherish yourself this week?

( ) Woke up restful most days   ( ) Meet daily water intake

( ) Went for short walk   ( ) Listen to favorite music

( ) Went for a long walk   ( ) Spent time with a loved one

( ) Practice mindful meditation   ( ) Pampered yourself

( ) Engaged in positive thinking   ( ) Read for pleasure

( ) Stretching / Yoga   ( ) Cooked a nourishing meal

( ) Worked out 3x or more   ( ) Practice gratitude

Add any additional self cherishes or health changes.

_____

_____

_____

_____

_____

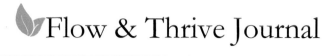Flow & Thrive Journal

Date
_____

I am capable, strong, and ready to take on the day.
Today, I choose joy, peace, and positivity in all I do.
_____

Today, I woke up and I appreciate it because:
_____
_____
_____
_____

Today, my health gratitude is:
_____
_____
_____
_____

Today, I discovered this about my health and/or self-care:
_____
_____
_____
_____

Today, was not a good day, and this is how I handled it:
_____
_____
_____
_____

FLOW & THRIVE
WEEKLY CHECKLIST

Journaling healthcare is a loving commitment to oneself.

How did you cherish yourself this week?

( ) Woke up restful most days   ( ) Meet daily water intake

( ) Went for short walk   ( ) Listen to favorite music

( ) Went for a long walk   ( ) Spent time with a loved one

( ) Practice mindful meditation   ( ) Pampered yourself

( ) Engaged in positive thinking   ( ) Read for pleasure

( ) Stretching / Yoga   ( ) Cooked a nourishing meal

( ) Worked out 3x or more   ( ) Practice gratitude

Add any additional self cherishes or health changes.

_____

_____

_____

_____

_____

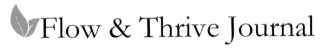# Flow & Thrive Journal

Date

_____

I am capable, strong, and ready to take on the day.
Today, I choose joy, peace, and positivity in all I do.

_____

Today, I woke up and I appreciate it because:

_____
_____
_____
_____

Today, my health gratitude is:

_____
_____
_____
_____

Today, I discovered this about my health and/or self-care:

_____
_____
_____
_____

Today, was not a good day, and this is how I handled it:

_____
_____
_____
_____

FLOW & THRIVE
WEEKLY CHECKLIST

Journaling healthcare is a loving commitment to oneself.

How did you cherish yourself this week?

( ) Woke up restful most days   ( ) Meet daily water intake

( ) Went for short walk   ( ) Listen to favorite music

( ) Went for a long walk   ( ) Spent time with a loved one

( ) Practice mindful meditation   ( ) Pampered yourself

( ) Engaged in positive thinking   ( ) Read for pleasure

( ) Stretching / Yoga   ( ) Cooked a nourishing meal

( ) Worked out 3x or more   ( ) Practice gratitude

Add any additional self cherishes or health changes.

_____

_____

_____

_____

_____

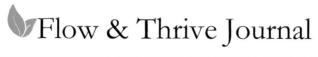Flow & Thrive Journal

Date
_____

_____

I am capable, strong, and ready to take on the day.
Today, I choose joy, peace, and positivity in all I do.

_____

Today, I woke up and I appreciate it because:

_____
_____
_____
_____

Today, my health gratitude is:

_____
_____
_____
_____

Today, I discovered this about my health and/or self-care:

_____
_____
_____
_____

Today, was not a good day, and this is how I handled it:

_____
_____
_____
_____

FLOW & THRIVE
WEEKLY CHECKLIST

Journaling healthcare is a loving commitment to oneself.

How did you cherish yourself this week?

( ) Woke up restful most days   ( ) Meet daily water intake

( ) Went for short walk   ( ) Listen to favorite music

( ) Went for a long walk   ( ) Spent time with a loved one

( ) Practice mindful meditation   ( ) Pampered yourself

( ) Engaged in positive thinking   ( ) Read for pleasure

( ) Stretching / Yoga   ( ) Cooked a nourishing meal

( ) Worked out 3x or more   ( ) Practice gratitude

Add any additional self cherishes or health changes.

_____

_____

_____

_____

_____

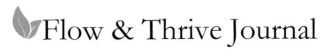Flow & Thrive Journal

Date
_____

I am capable, strong, and ready to take on the day.
Today, I choose joy, peace, and positivity in all I do.
_____

Today, I woke up and I appreciate it because:
_____
_____
_____
_____

Today, my health gratitude is:
_____
_____
_____
_____

Today, I discovered this about my health and/or self-care:
_____
_____
_____
_____

Today, was not a good day, and this is how I handled it:
_____
_____
_____
_____

FLOW & THRIVE
WEEKLY CHECKLIST

Journaling healthcare is a loving commitment to oneself.
How did you cherish yourself this week?

( ) Woke up restful most days   ( ) Meet daily water intake

( ) Went for short walk   ( ) Listen to favorite music

( ) Went for a long walk   ( ) Spent time with a loved one

( ) Practice mindful meditation   ( ) Pampered yourself

( ) Engaged in positive thinking   ( ) Read for pleasure

( ) Stretching / Yoga   ( ) Cooked a nourishing meal

( ) Worked out 3x or more   ( ) Practice gratitude

Add any additional self cherishes or health changes.

_____

_____

_____

_____

_____

_____

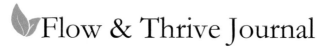Flow & Thrive Journal

Date

I am capable, strong, and ready to take on the day.
Today, I choose joy, peace, and positivity in all I do.

Today, I woke up and I appreciate it because:

_____
_____
_____
_____

Today, my health gratitude is:

_____
_____
_____
_____

Today, I discovered this about my health and/or self-care:

_____
_____
_____
_____

Today, was not a good day, and this is how I handled it:

_____
_____
_____
_____

FLOW & THRIVE
WEEKLY CHECKLIST

Journaling healthcare is a loving commitment to oneself.

How did you cherish yourself this week?

( ) Woke up restful most days   ( ) Meet daily water intake

( ) Went for short walk   ( ) Listen to favorite music

( ) Went for a long walk   ( ) Spent time with a loved one

( ) Practice mindful meditation   ( ) Pampered yourself

( ) Engaged in positive thinking ( ) Read for pleasure

( ) Stretching / Yoga   ( ) Cooked a nourishing meal

( ) Worked out 3x or more   ( ) Practice gratitude

Add any additional self cherishes or health changes.

_____

_____

_____

_____

_____

_____

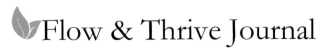Flow & Thrive Journal

Date

I am capable, strong, and ready to take on the day.
Today, I choose joy, peace, and positivity in all I do.

Today, I woke up and I appreciate it because:

_____
_____
_____
_____

Today, my health gratitude is:

_____
_____
_____
_____

Today, I discovered this about my health and/or self-care:

_____
_____
_____
_____

Today, was not a good day, and this is how I handled it:

_____
_____
_____
_____

FLOW & THRIVE
WEEKLY CHECKLIST

Journaling healthcare is a loving commitment to oneself.
How did you cherish yourself this week?

( ) Woke up restful most days   ( ) Meet daily water intake

( ) Went for short walk   ( ) Listen to favorite music

( ) Went for a long walk   ( ) Spent time with a loved one

( ) Practice mindful meditation   ( ) Pampered yourself

( ) Engaged in positive thinking   ( ) Read for pleasure

( ) Stretching / Yoga   ( ) Cooked a nourishing meal

( ) Worked out 3x or more   ( ) Practice gratitude

Add any additional self cherishes or health changes.

_____

_____

_____

_____

_____

_____

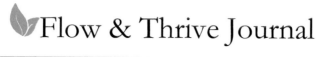 # Flow & Thrive Journal

Date
_____

I am capable, strong, and ready to take on the day.
Today, I choose joy, peace, and positivity in all I do.
_____

Today, I woke up and I appreciate it because:

_____
_____
_____
_____

Today, my health gratitude is:

_____
_____
_____
_____

Today, I discovered this about my health and/or self-care:

_____
_____
_____
_____

Today, was not a good day, and this is how I handled it:

_____
_____
_____
_____

FLOW & THRIVE
WEEKLY CHECKLIST

Journaling healthcare is a loving commitment to oneself.

How did you cherish yourself this week?

( ) Woke up restful most days   ( ) Meet daily water intake

( ) Went for short walk   ( ) Listen to favorite music

( ) Went for a long walk   ( ) Spent time with a loved one

( ) Practice mindful meditation   ( ) Pampered yourself

( ) Engaged in positive thinking   ( ) Read for pleasure

( ) Stretching / Yoga   ( ) Cooked a nourishing meal

( ) Worked out 3x or more   ( ) Practice gratitude

Add any additional self cherishes or health changes.

_____

_____

_____

_____

_____

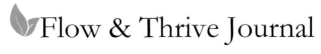Flow & Thrive Journal

Date
_____

I am capable, strong, and ready to take on the day.
Today, I choose joy, peace, and positivity in all I do.

Today, I woke up and I appreciate it because:
_____
_____
_____
_____

Today, my health gratitude is:
_____
_____
_____
_____

Today, I discovered this about my health and/or self-care:
_____
_____
_____
_____

Today, was not a good day, and this is how I handled it:
_____
_____
_____
_____

FLOW & THRIVE
WEEKLY CHECKLIST

Journaling healthcare is a loving commitment to oneself.
How did you cherish yourself this week?

( ) Woke up restful most days   ( ) Meet daily water intake

( ) Went for short walk   ( ) Listen to favorite music

( ) Went for a long walk   ( ) Spent time with a loved one

( ) Practice mindful meditation   ( ) Pampered yourself

( ) Engaged in positive thinking   ( ) Read for pleasure

( ) Stretching / Yoga   ( ) Cooked a nourishing meal

( ) Worked out 3x or more   ( ) Practice gratitude

Add any additional self cherishes or health changes.

_____

_____

_____

_____

_____

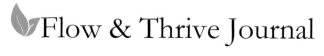

Flow & Thrive Journal

Date
_____

I am capable, strong, and ready to take on the day.
Today, I choose joy, peace, and positivity in all I do.
_____

Today, I woke up and I appreciate it because:
_____
_____
_____
_____

Today, my health gratitude is:
_____
_____
_____
_____

Today, I discovered this about my health and/or self-care:
_____
_____
_____
_____

Today, was not a good day, and this is how I handled it:
_____
_____
_____
_____

FLOW & THRIVE
WEEKLY CHECKLIST

Journaling healthcare is a loving commitment to oneself.
How did you cherish yourself this week?

( ) Woke up restful most days   ( ) Meet daily water intake

( ) Went for short walk   ( ) Listen to favorite music

( ) Went for a long walk   ( ) Spent time with a loved one

( ) Practice mindful meditation   ( ) Pampered yourself

( ) Engaged in positive thinking   ( ) Read for pleasure

( ) Stretching / Yoga   ( ) Cooked a nourishing meal

( ) Worked out 3x or more   ( ) Practice gratitude

Add any additional self cherishes or health changes.

_____

_____

_____

_____

_____

_____

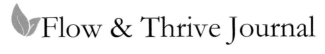Flow & Thrive Journal

Date
_____

I am capable, strong, and ready to take on the day.
Today, I choose joy, peace, and positivity in all I do.

Today, I woke up and I appreciate it because:
_____
_____
_____
_____

Today, my health gratitude is:
_____
_____
_____
_____

Today, I discovered this about my health and/or self-care:
_____
_____
_____
_____

Today, was not a good day, and this is how I handled it:
_____
_____
_____
_____

FLOW & THRIVE
WEEKLY CHECKLIST

Journaling healthcare is a loving commitment to oneself.
How did you cherish yourself this week?

( ) Woke up restful most days   ( ) Meet daily water intake

( ) Went for short walk   ( ) Listen to favorite music

( ) Went for a long walk   ( ) Spent time with a loved one

( ) Practice mindful meditation   ( ) Pampered yourself

( ) Engaged in positive thinking   ( ) Read for pleasure

( ) Stretching / Yoga   ( ) Cooked a nourishing meal

( ) Worked out 3x or more   ( ) Practice gratitude

Add any additional self cherishes or health changes.

_____

_____

_____

_____

_____

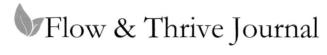

Flow & Thrive Journal

Date
_____

I am capable, strong, and ready to take on the day.
Today, I choose joy, peace, and positivity in all I do.
_____

Today, I woke up and I appreciate it because:
_____
_____
_____
_____

Today, my health gratitude is:
_____
_____
_____
_____

Today, I discovered this about my health and/or self-care:
_____
_____
_____
_____

Today, was not a good day, and this is how I handled it:
_____
_____
_____
_____

FLOW & THRIVE
WEEKLY CHECKLIST

Journaling healthcare is a loving commitment to oneself.

How did you cherish yourself this week?

( ) Woke up restful most days   ( ) Meet daily water intake

( ) Went for short walk   ( ) Listen to favorite music

( ) Went for a long walk   ( ) Spent time with a loved one

( ) Practice mindful meditation   ( ) Pampered yourself

( ) Engaged in positive thinking   ( ) Read for pleasure

( ) Stretching / Yoga   ( ) Cooked a nourishing meal

( ) Worked out 3x or more   ( ) Practice gratitude

Add any additional self cherishes or health changes.

_____

_____

_____

_____

_____

_____

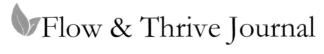Flow & Thrive Journal

Date
_____

I am capable, strong, and ready to take on the day.
Today, I choose joy, peace, and positivity in all I do.
_____

Today, I woke up and I appreciate it because:

_____
_____
_____
_____

Today, my health gratitude is:

_____
_____
_____
_____

Today, I discovered this about my health and/or self-care:

_____
_____
_____
_____

Today, was not a good day, and this is how I handled it:

_____
_____
_____
_____

FLOW & THRIVE
WEEKLY CHECKLIST

Journaling healthcare is a loving commitment to oneself.
How did you cherish yourself this week?

( ) Woke up restful most days   ( ) Meet daily water intake

( ) Went for short walk   ( ) Listen to favorite music

( ) Went for a long walk   ( ) Spent time with a loved one

( ) Practice mindful meditation   ( ) Pampered yourself

( ) Engaged in positive thinking   ( ) Read for pleasure

( ) Stretching / Yoga   ( ) Cooked a nourishing meal

( ) Worked out 3x or more   ( ) Practice gratitude

Add any additional self cherishes or health changes.

_____

_____

_____

_____

_____

_____

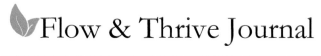# Flow & Thrive Journal

Date

_____

I am capable, strong, and ready to take on the day.
Today, I choose joy, peace, and positivity in all I do.

_____

Today, I woke up and I appreciate it because:

_____
_____
_____
_____

Today, my health gratitude is:

_____
_____
_____
_____

Today, I discovered this about my health and/or self-care:

_____
_____
_____
_____

Today, was not a good day, and this is how I handled it:

_____
_____
_____
_____

FLOW & THRIVE
WEEKLY CHECKLIST

Journaling healthcare is a loving commitment to oneself.
How did you cherish yourself this week?

( ) Woke up restful most days   ( ) Meet daily water intake

( ) Went for short walk   ( ) Listen to favorite music

( ) Went for a long walk   ( ) Spent time with a loved one

( ) Practice mindful meditation   ( ) Pampered yourself

( ) Engaged in positive thinking   ( ) Read for pleasure

( ) Stretching / Yoga   ( ) Cooked a nourishing meal

( ) Worked out 3x or more   ( ) Practice gratitude

Add any additional self cherishes or health changes.

_____

_____

_____

_____

_____

_____

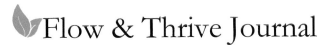

Flow & Thrive Journal

Date

_____

I am capable, strong, and ready to take on the day.
Today, I choose joy, peace, and positivity in all I do.

_____

Today, I woke up and I appreciate it because:

_____
_____
_____
_____

Today, my health gratitude is:

_____
_____
_____
_____

Today, I discovered this about my health and/or self-care:

_____
_____
_____
_____

Today, was not a good day, and this is how I handled it:

_____
_____
_____
_____

FLOW & THRIVE
WEEKLY CHECKLIST

Journaling healthcare is a loving commitment to oneself.
How did you cherish yourself this week?

( ) Woke up restful most days   ( ) Meet daily water intake

( ) Went for short walk   ( ) Listen to favorite music

( ) Went for a long walk   ( ) Spent time with a loved one

( ) Practice mindful meditation   ( ) Pampered yourself

( ) Engaged in positive thinking   ( ) Read for pleasure

( ) Stretching / Yoga   ( ) Cooked a nourishing meal

( ) Worked out 3x or more   ( ) Practice gratitude

Add any additional self cherishes or health changes.

_____

_____

_____

_____

_____

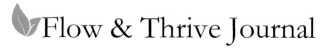# Flow & Thrive Journal

Date
_____

I am capable, strong, and ready to take on the day.
Today, I choose joy, peace, and positivity in all I do.
_____

Today, I woke up and I appreciate it because:
_____
_____
_____
_____

Today, my health gratitude is:
_____
_____
_____
_____

Today, I discovered this about my health and/or self-care:
_____
_____
_____
_____

Today, was not a good day, and this is how I handled it:
_____
_____
_____
_____

FLOW & THRIVE
WEEKLY CHECKLIST

Journaling healthcare is a loving commitment to oneself.

How did you cherish yourself this week?

- ( ) Woke up restful most days
- ( ) Went for short walk
- ( ) Went for a long walk
- ( ) Practice mindful meditation
- ( ) Engaged in positive thinking
- ( ) Stretching / Yoga
- ( ) Worked out 3x or more

- ( ) Meet daily water intake
- ( ) Listen to favorite music
- ( ) Spent time with a loved one
- ( ) Pampered yourself
- ( ) Read for pleasure
- ( ) Cooked a nourishing meal
- ( ) Practice gratitude

Add any additional self cherishes or health changes.

_____

_____

_____

_____

_____

_____

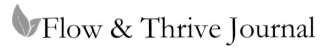Flow & Thrive Journal

Date
_____

I am capable, strong, and ready to take on the day.
Today, I choose joy, peace, and positivity in all I do.
_____

Today, I woke up and I appreciate it because:
_____
_____
_____
_____

Today, my health gratitude is:
_____
_____
_____
_____

Today, I discovered this about my health and/or self-care:
_____
_____
_____
_____

Today, was not a good day, and this is how I handled it:
_____
_____
_____
_____

FLOW & THRIVE
WEEKLY CHECKLIST

Journaling healthcare is a loving commitment to oneself.

How did you cherish yourself this week?

( ) Woke up restful most days   ( ) Meet daily water intake

( ) Went for short walk   ( ) Listen to favorite music

( ) Went for a long walk   ( ) Spent time with a loved one

( ) Practice mindful meditation   ( ) Pampered yourself

( ) Engaged in positive thinking   ( ) Read for pleasure

( ) Stretching / Yoga   ( ) Cooked a nourishing meal

( ) Worked out 3x or more   ( ) Practice gratitude

Add any additional self cherishes or health changes.

_____

_____

_____

_____

_____

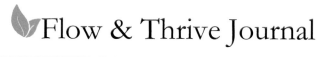# Flow & Thrive Journal

Date
_____

I am capable, strong, and ready to take on the day.
Today, I choose joy, peace, and positivity in all I do.

_____

Today, I woke up and I appreciate it because:

_____
_____
_____
_____

Today, my health gratitude is:

_____
_____
_____
_____

Today, I discovered this about my health and/or self-care:

_____
_____
_____
_____

Today, was not a good day, and this is how I handled it:

_____
_____
_____
_____

FLOW & THRIVE
WEEKLY CHECKLIST

Journaling healthcare is a loving commitment to oneself.
How did you cherish yourself this week?

( ) Woke up restful most days   ( ) Meet daily water intake

( ) Went for short walk   ( ) Listen to favorite music

( ) Went for a long walk   ( ) Spent time with a loved one

( ) Practice mindful meditation   ( ) Pampered yourself

( ) Engaged in positive thinking   ( ) Read for pleasure

( ) Stretching / Yoga   ( ) Cooked a nourishing meal

( ) Worked out 3x or more   ( ) Practice gratitude

Add any additional self cherishes or health changes.

_____

_____

_____

_____

_____

_____

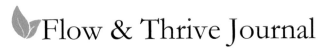Flow & Thrive Journal

Date

I am capable, strong, and ready to take on the day.
Today, I choose joy, peace, and positivity in all I do.

Today, I woke up and I appreciate it because:

_____

_____

_____

_____

Today, my health gratitude is:

_____

_____

_____

_____

Today, I discovered this about my health and/or self-care:

_____

_____

_____

_____

Today, was not a good day, and this is how I handled it:

_____

_____

_____

_____

FLOW & THRIVE
WEEKLY CHECKLIST

Journaling healthcare is a loving commitment to oneself.
How did you cherish yourself this week?

( ) Woke up restful most days   ( ) Meet daily water intake

( ) Went for short walk   ( ) Listen to favorite music

( ) Went for a long walk   ( ) Spent time with a loved one

( ) Practice mindful meditation   ( ) Pampered yourself

( ) Engaged in positive thinking   ( ) Read for pleasure

( ) Stretching / Yoga   ( ) Cooked a nourishing meal

( ) Worked out 3x or more   ( ) Practice gratitude

Add any additional self cherishes or health changes.

_____

_____

_____

_____

_____

_____

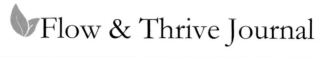Flow & Thrive Journal

Date
_____

I am capable, strong, and ready to take on the day.
Today, I choose joy, peace, and positivity in all I do.
_____

Today, I woke up and I appreciate it because:
_____
_____
_____
_____

Today, my health gratitude is:
_____
_____
_____
_____

Today, I discovered this about my health and/or self-care:
_____
_____
_____
_____

Today, was not a good day, and this is how I handled it:
_____
_____
_____
_____

FLOW & THRIVE
WEEKLY CHECKLIST

Journaling healthcare is a loving commitment to oneself.

How did you cherish yourself this week?

( ) Woke up restful most days   ( ) Meet daily water intake

( ) Went for short walk   ( ) Listen to favorite music

( ) Went for a long walk   ( ) Spent time with a loved one

( ) Practice mindful meditation   ( ) Pampered yourself

( ) Engaged in positive thinking   ( ) Read for pleasure

( ) Stretching / Yoga   ( ) Cooked a nourishing meal

( ) Worked out 3x or more   ( ) Practice gratitude

Add any additional self cherishes or health changes.

_____

_____

_____

_____

_____

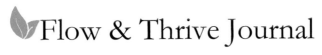Flow & Thrive Journal

Date

_____

I am capable, strong, and ready to take on the day.
Today, I choose joy, peace, and positivity in all I do.

_____

Today, I woke up and I appreciate it because:

_____

_____

_____

_____

Today, my health gratitude is:

_____

_____

_____

_____

Today, I discovered this about my health and/or self-care:

_____

_____

_____

_____

Today, was not a good day, and this is how I handled it:

_____

_____

_____

_____

FLOW & THRIVE
WEEKLY CHECKLIST

Journaling healthcare is a loving commitment to oneself.
How did you cherish yourself this week?

( ) Woke up restful most days   ( ) Meet daily water intake

( ) Went for short walk   ( ) Listen to favorite music

( ) Went for a long walk   ( ) Spent time with a loved one

( ) Practice mindful meditation   ( ) Pampered yourself

( ) Engaged in positive thinking   ( ) Read for pleasure

( ) Stretching / Yoga   ( ) Cooked a nourishing meal

( ) Worked out 3x or more   ( ) Practice gratitude

Add any additional self cherishes or health changes.

_____

_____

_____

_____

_____

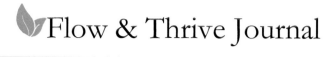
Flow & Thrive Journal

Date

I am capable, strong, and ready to take on the day.
Today, I choose joy, peace, and positivity in all I do.

Today, I woke up and I appreciate it because:

_____
_____
_____
_____

Today, my health gratitude is:

_____
_____
_____
_____

Today, I discovered this about my health and/or self-care:

_____
_____
_____
_____

Today, was not a good day, and this is how I handled it:

_____
_____
_____
_____

FLOW & THRIVE
WEEKLY CHECKLIST

Journaling healthcare is a loving commitment to oneself.

How did you cherish yourself this week?

( ) Woke up restful most days   ( ) Meet daily water intake

( ) Went for short walk   ( ) Listen to favorite music

( ) Went for a long walk   ( ) Spent time with a loved one

( ) Practice mindful meditation   ( ) Pampered yourself

( ) Engaged in positive thinking   ( ) Read for pleasure

( ) Stretching / Yoga   ( ) Cooked a nourishing meal

( ) Worked out 3x or more   ( ) Practice gratitude

Add any additional self cherishes or health changes.

_____

_____

_____

_____

_____

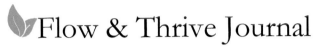Flow & Thrive Journal

Date
_____

I am capable, strong, and ready to take on the day.
Today, I choose joy, peace, and positivity in all I do.

Today, I woke up and I appreciate it because:
_____
_____
_____
_____

Today, my health gratitude is:
_____
_____
_____
_____

Today, I discovered this about my health and/or self-care:
_____
_____
_____
_____

Today, was not a good day, and this is how I handled it:
_____
_____
_____
_____

FLOW & THRIVE
WEEKLY CHECKLIST

Journaling healthcare is a loving commitment to oneself.
How did you cherish yourself this week?

( ) Woke up restful most days   ( ) Meet daily water intake

( ) Went for short walk   ( ) Listen to favorite music

( ) Went for a long walk   ( ) Spent time with a loved one

( ) Practice mindful meditation   ( ) Pampered yourself

( ) Engaged in positive thinking   ( ) Read for pleasure

( ) Stretching / Yoga   ( ) Cooked a nourishing meal

( ) Worked out 3x or more   ( ) Practice gratitude

Add any additional self cherishes or health changes.

_____

_____

_____

_____

_____

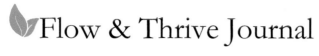Flow & Thrive Journal

Date

I am capable, strong, and ready to take on the day.
Today, I choose joy, peace, and positivity in all I do.

Today, I woke up and I appreciate it because:

_____
_____
_____
_____

Today, my health gratitude is:

_____
_____
_____
_____

Today, I discovered this about my health and/or self-care:

_____
_____
_____
_____

Today, was not a good day, and this is how I handled it:

_____
_____
_____
_____

FLOW & THRIVE
WEEKLY CHECKLIST

Journaling healthcare is a loving commitment to oneself.

How did you cherish yourself this week?

- ( ) Woke up restful most days
- ( ) Went for short walk
- ( ) Went for a long walk
- ( ) Practice mindful meditation
- ( ) Engaged in positive thinking
- ( ) Stretching / Yoga
- ( ) Worked out 3x or more

- ( ) Meet daily water intake
- ( ) Listen to favorite music
- ( ) Spent time with a loved one
- ( ) Pampered yourself
- ( ) Read for pleasure
- ( ) Cooked a nourishing meal
- ( ) Practice gratitude

Add any additional self cherishes or health changes.

_____

_____

_____

_____

_____

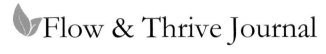Flow & Thrive Journal

Date
_____

I am capable, strong, and ready to take on the day.
Today, I choose joy, peace, and positivity in all I do.
_____

Today, I woke up and I appreciate it because:
_____
_____
_____
_____

Today, my health gratitude is:
_____
_____
_____
_____

Today, I discovered this about my health and/or self-care:
_____
_____
_____
_____

Today, was not a good day, and this is how I handled it:
_____
_____
_____
_____

FLOW & THRIVE
WEEKLY CHECKLIST

Journaling healthcare is a loving commitment to oneself.
How did you cherish yourself this week?

( ) Woke up restful most days   ( ) Meet daily water intake

( ) Went for short walk   ( ) Listen to favorite music

( ) Went for a long walk   ( ) Spent time with a loved one

( ) Practice mindful meditation   ( ) Pampered yourself

( ) Engaged in positive thinking   ( ) Read for pleasure

( ) Stretching / Yoga   ( ) Cooked a nourishing meal

( ) Worked out 3x or more   ( ) Practice gratitude

Add any additional self cherishes or health changes.

_____

_____

_____

_____

_____

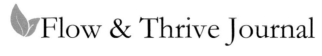

Flow & Thrive Journal

Date
_____

I am capable, strong, and ready to take on the day.
Today, I choose joy, peace, and positivity in all I do.
_____

Today, I woke up and I appreciate it because:

_____
_____
_____
_____

Today, my health gratitude is:

_____
_____
_____
_____

Today, I discovered this about my health and/or self-care:

_____
_____
_____
_____

Today, was not a good day, and this is how I handled it:

_____
_____
_____
_____

FLOW & THRIVE
WEEKLY CHECKLIST

Journaling healthcare is a loving commitment to oneself.

How did you cherish yourself this week?

( ) Woke up restful most days   ( ) Meet daily water intake

( ) Went for short walk   ( ) Listen to favorite music

( ) Went for a long walk   ( ) Spent time with a loved one

( ) Practice mindful meditation   ( ) Pampered yourself

( ) Engaged in positive thinking   ( ) Read for pleasure

( ) Stretching / Yoga   ( ) Cooked a nourishing meal

( ) Worked out 3x or more   ( ) Practice gratitude

Add any additional self cherishes or health changes.

_____

_____

_____

_____

_____

_____

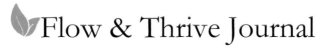Flow & Thrive Journal

Date
_____

I am capable, strong, and ready to take on the day.
Today, I choose joy, peace, and positivity in all I do.
_____

Today, I woke up and I appreciate it because:
_____
_____
_____
_____

Today, my health gratitude is:
_____
_____
_____
_____

Today, I discovered this about my health and/or self-care:
_____
_____
_____
_____

Today, was not a good day, and this is how I handled it:
_____
_____
_____
_____

FLOW & THRIVE
WEEKLY CHECKLIST

Journaling healthcare is a loving commitment to oneself.

How did you cherish yourself this week?

( ) Woke up restful most days   ( ) Meet daily water intake

( ) Went for short walk   ( ) Listen to favorite music

( ) Went for a long walk   ( ) Spent time with a loved one

( ) Practice mindful meditation   ( ) Pampered yourself

( ) Engaged in positive thinking   ( ) Read for pleasure

( ) Stretching / Yoga   ( ) Cooked a nourishing meal

( ) Worked out 3x or more   ( ) Practice gratitude

Add any additional self cherishes or health changes.

_____

_____

_____

_____

_____

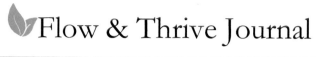Flow & Thrive Journal

Date

I am capable, strong, and ready to take on the day.
Today, I choose joy, peace, and positivity in all I do.

Today, I woke up and I appreciate it because:

_____

_____

_____

_____

Today, my health gratitude is:

_____

_____

_____

_____

Today, I discovered this about my health and/or self-care:

_____

_____

_____

_____

Today, was not a good day, and this is how I handled it:

_____

_____

_____

_____

FLOW & THRIVE
WEEKLY CHECKLIST

Journaling healthcare is a loving commitment to oneself.

How did you cherish yourself this week?

( ) Woke up restful most days ( ) Meet daily water intake

( ) Went for short walk   ( ) Listen to favorite music

( ) Went for a long walk   ( ) Spent time with a loved one

( ) Practice mindful meditation ( ) Pampered yourself

( ) Engaged in positive thinking ( ) Read for pleasure

( ) Stretching / Yoga   ( ) Cooked a nourishing meal

( ) Worked out 3x or more   ( ) Practice gratitude

Add any additional self cherishes or health changes.

_____

_____

_____

_____

_____

_____

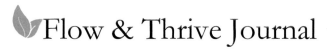# Flow & Thrive Journal

Date
_____

I am capable, strong, and ready to take on the day.
Today, I choose joy, peace, and positivity in all I do.

_____

Today, I woke up and I appreciate it because:

_____
_____
_____
_____

Today, my health gratitude is:

_____
_____
_____
_____

Today, I discovered this about my health and/or self-care:

_____
_____
_____
_____

Today, was not a good day, and this is how I handled it:

_____
_____
_____
_____

FLOW & THRIVE
WEEKLY CHECKLIST

Journaling healthcare is a loving commitment to oneself.
How did you cherish yourself this week?

( ) Woke up restful most days   ( ) Meet daily water intake

( ) Went for short walk   ( ) Listen to favorite music

( ) Went for a long walk   ( ) Spent time with a loved one

( ) Practice mindful meditation   ( ) Pampered yourself

( ) Engaged in positive thinking   ( ) Read for pleasure

( ) Stretching /Yoga   ( ) Cooked a nourishing meal

( ) Worked out 3x or more   ( ) Practice gratitude

Add any additional self cherishes or health changes.

_____

_____

_____

_____

_____

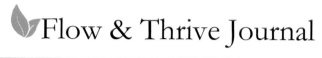Flow & Thrive Journal

Date
_____

I am capable, strong, and ready to take on the day.
Today, I choose joy, peace, and positivity in all I do.

_____

Today, I woke up and I appreciate it because:
_____
_____
_____
_____

Today, my health gratitude is:
_____
_____
_____
_____

Today, I discovered this about my health and/or self-care:
_____
_____
_____
_____

Today, was not a good day, and this is how I handled it:
_____
_____
_____
_____

FLOW & THRIVE
WEEKLY CHECKLIST

Journaling healthcare is a loving commitment to oneself.
How did you cherish yourself this week?

( ) Woke up restful most days   ( ) Meet daily water intake

( ) Went for short walk   ( ) Listen to favorite music

( ) Went for a long walk   ( ) Spent time with a loved one

( ) Practice mindful meditation   ( ) Pampered yourself

( ) Engaged in positive thinking   ( ) Read for pleasure

( ) Stretching / Yoga   ( ) Cooked a nourishing meal

( ) Worked out 3x or more   ( ) Practice gratitude

Add any additional self cherishes or health changes.

_____

_____

_____

_____

_____

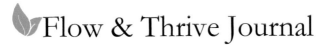Flow & Thrive Journal

Date
_____

I am capable, strong, and ready to take on the day.
Today, I choose joy, peace, and positivity in all I do.
_____

Today, I woke up and I appreciate it because:
_____
_____
_____
_____

Today, my health gratitude is:
_____
_____
_____
_____

Today, I discovered this about my health and/or self-care:
_____
_____
_____
_____

Today, was not a good day, and this is how I handled it:
_____
_____
_____
_____

FLOW & THRIVE
WEEKLY CHECKLIST

Journaling healthcare is a loving commitment to oneself.

How did you cherish yourself this week?

( ) Woke up restful most days   ( ) Meet daily water intake

( ) Went for short walk   ( ) Listen to favorite music

( ) Went for a long walk   ( ) Spent time with a loved one

( ) Practice mindful meditation   ( ) Pampered yourself

( ) Engaged in positive thinking   ( ) Read for pleasure

( ) Stretching / Yoga   ( ) Cooked a nourishing meal

( ) Worked out 3x or more   ( ) Practice gratitude

Add any additional self cherishes or health changes.

_____

_____

_____

_____

_____

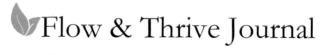Flow & Thrive Journal

Date
_____

I am capable, strong, and ready to take on the day.
Today, I choose joy, peace, and positivity in all I do.

_____

Today, I woke up and I appreciate it because:
_____
_____
_____
_____

Today, my health gratitude is:
_____
_____
_____
_____

Today, I discovered this about my health and/or self-care:
_____
_____
_____
_____

Today, was not a good day, and this is how I handled it:
_____
_____
_____
_____

FLOW & THRIVE
WEEKLY CHECKLIST

Journaling healthcare is a loving commitment to oneself.

How did you cherish yourself this week?

( ) Woke up restful most days   ( ) Meet daily water intake

( ) Went for short walk   ( ) Listen to favorite music

( ) Went for a long walk   ( ) Spent time with a loved one

( ) Practice mindful meditation   ( ) Pampered yourself

( ) Engaged in positive thinking   ( ) Read for pleasure

( ) Stretching / Yoga   ( ) Cooked a nourishing meal

( ) Worked out 3x or more   ( ) Practice gratitude

Add any additional self cherishes or health changes.

_____

_____

_____

_____

_____

_____

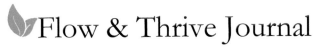Flow & Thrive Journal

Date
_____

I am capable, strong, and ready to take on the day.
Today, I choose joy, peace, and positivity in all I do.

_____

Today, I woke up and I appreciate it because:
_____
_____
_____
_____

Today, my health gratitude is:
_____
_____
_____
_____

Today, I discovered this about my health and/or self-care:
_____
_____
_____
_____

Today, was not a good day, and this is how I handled it:
_____
_____
_____
_____

FLOW & THRIVE
WEEKLY CHECKLIST

Journaling healthcare is a loving commitment to oneself.

How did you cherish yourself this week?

( ) Woke up restful most days

( ) Went for short walk

( ) Went for a long walk

( ) Practice mindful meditation

( ) Engaged in positive thinking

( ) Stretching / Yoga

( ) Worked out 3x or more

( ) Meet daily water intake

( ) Listen to favorite music

( ) Spent time with a loved one

( ) Pampered yourself

( ) Read for pleasure

( ) Cooked a nourishing meal

( ) Practice gratitude

Add any additional self cherishes or health changes.

_____

_____

_____

_____

_____

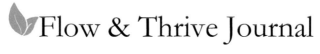Flow & Thrive Journal

Date
_____

I am capable, strong, and ready to take on the day.
Today, I choose joy, peace, and positivity in all I do.

Today, I woke up and I appreciate it because:

_____
_____
_____
_____

Today, my health gratitude is:

_____
_____
_____
_____

Today, I discovered this about my health and/or self-care:

_____
_____
_____
_____

Today, was not a good day, and this is how I handled it:

_____
_____
_____
_____

FLOW & THRIVE
WEEKLY CHECKLIST

Journaling healthcare is a loving commitment to oneself.

How did you cherish yourself this week?

( ) Woke up restful most days   ( ) Meet daily water intake

( ) Went for short walk   ( ) Listen to favorite music

( ) Went for a long walk   ( ) Spent time with a loved one

( ) Practice mindful meditation   ( ) Pampered yourself

( ) Engaged in positive thinking   ( ) Read for pleasure

( ) Stretching / Yoga   ( ) Cooked a nourishing meal

( ) Worked out 3x or more   ( ) Practice gratitude

Add any additional self cherishes or health changes.

_____

_____

_____

_____

_____

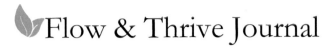# Flow & Thrive Journal

Date
_____

I am capable, strong, and ready to take on the day.
Today, I choose joy, peace, and positivity in all I do.
_____

Today, I woke up and I appreciate it because:
_____
_____
_____
_____

Today, my health gratitude is:
_____
_____
_____
_____

Today, I discovered this about my health and/or self-care:
_____
_____
_____
_____

Today, was not a good day, and this is how I handled it:
_____
_____
_____
_____

FLOW & THRIVE
WEEKLY CHECKLIST

Journaling healthcare is a loving commitment to oneself.

How did you cherish yourself this week?

( ) Woke up restful most days   ( ) Meet daily water intake

( ) Went for short walk   ( ) Listen to favorite music

( ) Went for a long walk   ( ) Spent time with a loved one

( ) Practice mindful meditation   ( ) Pampered yourself

( ) Engaged in positive thinking   ( ) Read for pleasure

( ) Stretching /Yoga   ( ) Cooked a nourishing meal

( ) Worked out 3x or more   ( ) Practice gratitude

Add any additional self cherishes or health changes.

_____

_____

_____

_____

_____

_____

Made in the USA
Columbia, SC
27 November 2024

47766885R00097